God and Gerson Therapy:
Diary of a Cancer Patient

Lynn Ford

Copyright © 2014 Lynn Ford

All rights reserved.

ISBN-10: 1495257304
ISBN-13: 9781495257308

Acknowledgements

I want to first thank God for so clearly orchestrating the events of my life in such a way as I could see and feel, these past 14 months. Here, I acknowledge not only those who have helped inspire the writings in this book, but those who have lifted my soul, met my physical needs and drenched me in love and emotional support since my cancer diagnosis in December of 2012. I want to thank my Mom, Janet Ford for working in the kitchen tirelessly EVERY day for the 8 months I have been practicing Gerson therapy. You deserve a medal. I want to thank my sister Shelley Loring, cousin Lisa Peters and brothers, Mark and Steven Ford for their continued support, as well as the support and prayers of other family members. I want to extend my gratitude for my Christian family of the Boston Church of Christ and Christ Community Church of Providence as well as many spiritual brothers and sisters worldwide sending prayers and well wishes. I am grateful for those who drove me to all my surgeries and appointments; Vivi, Steve, Lori, Amy, Shelley, Mark, Beti and Angela. Thank you Anne Hannon for being the loudest fan of my writing and encouraging me to publish. Thank you Suzette Standring for your input and promotion. A special thanks goes to my boss Madelyn D'Addario for holding down the fort and freeing me up to do what I needed to do. I am grateful for all the support my team and ALL my co-workers poured out for me during this challenging time. A special thanks also goes to Amy Oliveira for proof reading for me and getting me to yoga each week. Bless you! Thank you Beth Buccholz and June Smith for going the extra mile for me when I embarked on Gerson therapy and for your words of support even if you weren't quite sure it would work. I also owe so much to Amelia Chaves Ferro, Janice Wellington, Juanita Land and Bronwyn Planchard for being there during my time of learning in CA and to Dr. Donald Stillings and Janet Stillings of The Longevity Center for sharing your knowledge of Gerson therapy with me.

I am grateful for the men who penned the scriptures that give me life each day. All the scriptures quoted in the pages to follow are taken from the 2011 edition of the New International Version Bible.

Cover photos are by Lisa Fischer at lisafischerphotography.com. Perfect, Lisa, thanks!

Table of Contents

Acknowledgements iii
Introduction vii
Part One: Making the Gerson Therapy Discovery 1
    Yes, science determines everything, but I often fail to recognize that God is the scientist.
Part Two: Turning to Gerson in Desperation 41
    I'm fighting to hold the line. I'm pushing hard to gain a hair line, a fraction of a millimeter.
Part Three: The Honeymoon is Over 101
    Yesterday I was dozing off on the bathroom floor or as I call it, 'the coffee lounge.'
Part Four: Living Victoriously! 141
    I see Him! Do you see Him?
In Conclusion 185
Other Purported Cancer Fighters .187
Favorite Books, Documentaries and Juicers. 189

Introduction

My name is Lynn Ford. When I was 51 years old, in December of 2012, I was diagnosed with bladder cancer. I underwent surgery to remove a tumor the size of a golf ball and then underwent 6 weeks of something called BCG treatment. During this treatment, a TB virus (of sorts) was inserted into my bladder, I held it for two hours and then released it. This BCG was supposed to stimulate my immune system. After the 6 weeks we waited another month for my bladder to heal and then I went in for biopsy surgery in April. Not only was the cancer back, but in many new places in my bladder. The BCG had failed. My urologist said he would have to take my bladder out and in a hurry before the cancer spread outside the bladder. He said this was high grade cancer, another round of BCG would not work and surgery had to be immanent. It was a scary conversation. The scariest conversation I have ever had in my life. I wasn't sure what to do.

At first, I was pretty resigned to let him take my bladder out, but after a few more days I thought, "There's got to be a better way." I had watched 3 Gerson therapy documentaries and read half the book, *Healing the Gerson Way*, by Charlotte Gerson and Beata Bishop. The claims of healing were unbelievable. The case studies were compelling. The testimonies I had seen in the videos were convincing. Even so, I thought I didn't have time. How could I just pick up and go to a place I could learn Gerson therapy? Surely, it was too late. Even if Gerson therapy worked, how much would I need to tip the scales in my favor?

I went to another doctor for a second opinion. He said we could give BCG another try. In my heart I knew another round of BCG without Gerson would not work, but just his saying to give it another try, gave me the confidence to take a chance on Gerson. I also feel strongly that God was setting me up for success, since I had been moved to radically change my lifestyle and diet 4 months prior to my diagnosis.

I flew to California and spent 10 days learning and practicing Gerson therapy under the care of Dr. Donald Stillings and his wife Janet. On May 22nd I had another surgery to clean out my bladder. I had another round of BCG accompanied with strict adherence to Gerson therapy plus plenty of rest, no work. On Sept 4th I had biopsy surgery which revealed that all the cancer, the high grade cancer, was gone. That's my story! And to me, it is an amazing story that I never tire of. Now, I must continue Gerson therapy until 2 years are complete to make sure all the toxicity is out and the cancer does not return.

Writing has helped me to stay on task. On December 16th of 2012, I began posting entries on Caring Bridge, a website designed for seriously ill people and their families to post information about the patient so friends and family can be kept abreast of the patient's status. It soon became evident that the daily posts were more like a diary entry for me than purely informational. Then, even if I didn't have any important news or updates, I tried to post something every day because I knew some folks would be waiting for my next update. In October of 2013, I started a Facebook blog called, "Gerson Girl." In the pages that follow are many days of my journey. I also understand that if you are purchasing this book, you may be in a panicked mode, hungry for information to help you make a difficult decision on a short time table. With that in mind, I will supply, first, critical information that you may be looking for right this minute. Welcome to the amazing world of Gerson therapy! Love to you, Lynn

What You Need to Know Now

There are a few reasons you might have purchased this book. You have heard of Gerson therapy or know someone on Gerson therapy and are intrigued and want to learn more. Maybe, you have a serious illness, a chronic, debilitating illness and you wonder if Gerson is something you might want to do. Or you or someone close to you is very seriously ill and is being pressed to make life altering decisions that could heal and give life or fail and leave you worse than when you started. Unfortunately, all too often, patients find themselves staring at a doctor who is telling them they need to do such and such, right away or things might go really bad and the patient has no knowledge whatsoever what their options really are.

Patients, trusting doctors to know all, quickly surrender to the doctor's prescription for surgery, chemo or other drugs that can do incredible damage to the body. Please educate yourself on Gerson therapy before saying yes to anything! I found myself in just this position and luckily, I had already begun to learn about Gerson and already had faith that it worked and could work for me.

First of all, if you are in a state where you NEED information FAST and you have not read, *Healing the Gerson Way*, drop this book, call your nearest bookstore, ask them if they carry, *Healing the Gerson Way*, pick it up straight away and sit down and devour it. If they do not have it, jump on line and order it or check out the library. It is critical that you get the most complete package of information you can get to help you make the tough decisions you need to make about your treatment plans. This book is more about getting through Gerson therapy after you have decided to jump in the water. However, if you are already considering Gerson therapy and you just don't know if you can do it, this book can help give you the confidence to make the commitment. It is also a great introduction to friends or family who have serious illness to give them the chance to choose Gerson for themselves.

What is Gerson Therapy?

Max Gerson MD was a doctor who lived and practiced in Germany as far back as the 1920s. Because of his own struggle with migraine headaches, he began experimenting with different foods to see if he could cure himself. He had a theory that most disease was caused by two problems: nutritional deficiency and toxicity. The answer, he thought, must be hyper alimentation (hyper-nutrition) and detoxification. He addressed deficiency with fresh pressed juices, orange, green, carrot and carrot and apple combined, up to 13 eight ounce drinks a day. And to address the toxicity he used coffee enemas, up to 5 a day, to keep toxins moving out of the body and, vitally important, to protect the liver. In addition, the diet he prescribes is very limiting: ALL organic, veggies and fruit, some raw, some cooked; oatmeal in the morning; a slice of organic rye bread, no oils except flax seed oil. There is not allowed animal products of any kind, including meat and dairy. That's right, no eggs, no yogurt, no milk, no ICE CREAM! There is no fish or pork or chicken. There is not allowed beans, nuts and seeds, other oils and all processed foods. Also, water must be distilled. YIKES! Yeah, you ain't kiddin'! The absolutely

AMAZING thing is, when you start on this therapy your body begins to heal VERY quickly.

Max Gerson discovered that doing this very tough regimen, he was able to cure himself of migraines. He then healed a girl of her migraines, but also discovered that her incurable TB was cured. He then cured over 400 TB patients using this therapy. And what he quickly realized was that when you heal the body the body will heal disease. He hadn't developed a therapy for migraines or TB or cancer, for that matter. He developed a way for the body to restore all its own healing abilities to handle almost ALL disease. WOW! Amazing!!

Well? If this is so, why is there any disease left at all? Why didn't my grandfather know this or my mother? The fact is that Max Gerson was a highly respected doctor in Germany. Because of the Nazi threat, he moved to the US with his family where he had a thriving medical practice in New York. He was using this same therapy to heal cancer patients, patients often that had been sent home to die. In 1946, Max Gerson went before a congressional committee and presented 5 of his healed patients and their medical records and stated that he had healed his patients with this therapy. The powers that be, calling him a quack, black balled him and made it impossible for him to continue his work in New York. Even the newscaster, who announced on TV that Gerson had found the cure for cancer, was fired shortly after the broadcast, after being with NBC for 30 years. Apparently, it is illegal in the US, if you are an MD to claim you can cure cancer with any measure other than what the powerful licensing authorities say. And you can lose your license if you claim otherwise or practice otherwise. Hmmm.

Gerson opened a Gerson Hospital in Tijuana, Mexico. It is still there and still thriving. Max Gerson died when he was in his 80's of arsenic poisoning. There is also a Gerson hospital in Hungry. There was one in Fukushima, Japan. I am not sure of the status of that hospital since the nuclear meltdown there. I believe there is one in Spain. There are also places you can find on line to go and learn this therapy or if you need to, you can try doing it simply by reading the book. Obviously, the more knowledge and the more knowledgeable people you can have around you, the more likely your success.

What Gerson Therapy Can't Do?

As listed in, *Healing the Gerson Way,* diseases difficult, but possible, to cure with Gerson therapy are brain cancer because of inflammation in the brain during the healing process; bone metastases because of the pain and the patience needed to stick with the therapy; open breast cancer lesions; multiple myeloma; long-term prednisone and/or chemotherapy treatment. There are other diseases that just don't respond to Gerson therapy. These include: amyotrophic lateral sclerosis (ALS), Parkinson's disease, chronic kidney disease, emphysema and muscular dystrophy.

What are the nuts and bolts really?

How fast can Gerson start to heal?

The answer is simply, the day you begin. The first 3 months are critical to beating the progression of an aggressive disease. The official length of therapy is a full 2 years and should not be stopped prior to 2 years even though all symptoms and evidence of disease will be most likely be gone much earlier in the treatment. I was on Gerson therapy, along with medical treatment (not chemo) for 4 months before my biopsy revealed the high grade cancer was gone.

How quickly can I learn to do the therapy?

You can learn in a few days. I, of course, think that seeking training at a facility somewhere is the best way to learn so that you don't miss anything and even more importantly, so that you will have the confidence that is critical to embark on this journey. I was tentative before I visited Dr. Stillings, but 10 days with him and I was ready to go. The details of the therapy are not as difficult to learn as wrapping your emotions and mind around the constant and demanding nature of the therapy.

Does insurance pay for Gerson therapy?

Unfortunately, the answer is no. Because I was receiving medical treatments at the same time I began Gerson therapy I was able to be covered by Short

Term Disability to cover my wages from my work. And luckily, the Short Term Disability also covered my time at The Longevity Center, where I learned how to do Gerson therapy. Once my medical treatments were over, Short Term Disability would not cover wages so that I could practice Gerson at home. Short Term Disability only covers time away from work if I am regularly seeing a medical professional and receiving procedures of some sort for the treatment of my cancer.

How much will this cost me?

The biggest variable will be how you choose to learn the therapy. If you are flat broke and all you can do is read, *Healing the Gerson Way*, then do it. You can also purchase on line programs from the Gerson Institute. You can attend a Gerson Institute workshop in person in CA, you can go to a Gerson Hospital in Tijuana or Hungary, the Charlotte Gerson Health Restoration Center in CA or one of the other non-Gerson certified facilities in the US, which you can find on line by Googling, "Gerson Therapy." After you have learned the therapy, the cost is pretty consistently predictable. I started in May of 2012 and the cost is roughly $200 a week for food, supplements and coffee. You may incur additional costs if you have to hire someone to come into your home to assist you either juicing or cooking or both. I was able to be at home for the first 3 months of my therapy so I could do most everything myself. My 81 year old mother has been helping a lot since my return to work. We spilt the chores and can get it all done. The good news is as the therapy progresses, the supplements are reduced a little bit, more and more.

However, in addition to the initial training cost, the food, supplements and coffee; there are also appliances needed for the therapy. Primarily, the juicer is the most critical piece of equipment in your operation. Max Gerson used a Norwalk and the Gerson Institute heavily promotes the use of this juicer. The challenge is the cost. I paid $2400.00 for my Norwalk. I used the Norwalk for 3 months. When I went back to work, I realized I could not continue because of the time it takes to operate. The Norwalk ensures that enzymes are not being heated and thus killed in the juicing process. It also ensures that you are getting more juice from your food than most any other juicer on the planet, saving money in the long run. I just want to give you an important note here if you choose to go with the Norwalk. I spent weeks trying to perfect using this machine without the hydraulic press spraying me with orange or green pulp. I thought I was putting too much pulp in the press cloth. Then I thought the cloth was misshapen by use and I needed to replace the cloth. Then I thought that I must not be folding the cloth correctly. The truth was, I was using a speed on the press that was far too fast. Once I slowed down the speed of the press, it politely stopped spraying me and the rest of the kitchen with pulp! When the Fusion came on the market, the makers of that machine also claimed to preserve the live enzymes in the juicing process. This juicer is superfast and does waste more food, but cost me only about $120.00. I have been using this juicer since the 3 month mark. Of course there are 100s of juicers to choose from, but it is essential that you have a juicer that maintains the living enzymes.

The therapy also requires that you use distilled water for all cooking and coffee enemas. You can buy distilled water by the gallon, but that lugging from the car will get old really fast. I purchased a Waterwise distiller for about $465.00. It sits on the counter top and a great by product of the water distiller is that it generates lots of heat. It can help keep the kitchen cozy in the winter. I've made other purchases which are not needed for the therapy, but that I thought would enhance my treatment. I purchased an infrared sauna to help detox. I bought a couple air purifiers. I bought a couple cooking appliances in order to save on the electric bill.

How much time does Gerson therapy take?

As I mentioned, the length of the therapy for cancer patients is a full 2 years. When I started, I thought it would be ok to skip days that I also had medical treatment on, which was 1 day a week. I quickly changed my mind. I would get headaches if I stopped. I can't say for sure if the headaches were related to the break in therapy, but they seemed to stop when I stopped taking days off. And why would you want to take days off anyway, only delaying your healing? The answer to that gets back to being emotionally tough with yourself. Don't be soft on yourself. Also, I wanted to give my Mom a break. Don't give into that defeating kind of thinking.

Okay, let's see how much time? The coffee enema is about 15 minutes on paper, but I have found that I actually need to do a quick water enema before each coffee enema. I have to transport coffee and water to the upstairs bathroom and now that it is cold here in New England, I need to heat the coffee and water for a few minutes. The bottom line is that 3 coffee enemas take me 1 and a half hours each day, 30 minutes each. I can do one before I go to work, one at about 4:30 after work and one at about 8:30, before bed. It takes about 20 minutes to cook the coffee and strain it into Mason jars.

In addition to juicing and taking enemas, there are other tasks. It might take 30 minutes a day to tend to the water distiller, making 3 gallons of water. I do not use a microwave so cooking anything takes 20 minutes or more. Heating food takes 5 or more minutes. At this point shopping is pretty straight forward and takes maybe an hour or a little more each week. Added all up, I am adding 3 to 3.5 hours onto each day. That is a lot if you have to work full time or take care of other family members.

Juicing starts with the shopping. When I have everything I need on hand, I have to prep and rinse greens for 3 green drinks. This takes maybe 10 or 15 minutes. Then I have to clean and cut 5 pounds of carrots. This takes 15 minutes. I then need to cut 3 apples. With the Fusion, I actually don't need to cut the apples, but Mom likes to take the seeds and stem out. It takes only a minute or so to actually make the drink in the Fusion. It takes a lot longer in the Norwalk. The time cleaning the Fusion is longer than the time to make a drink. Therefore, we only run the machine in the morning and clean it as soon as I have had 3 green drinks, which I can do in about 2 hours. It probably takes 10 minutes to clean the machine (or 40 minutes if you are my Mom.)

What are other hidden costs to count?

If you are adding 3 hours onto your already busy day then you have to also give up whatever currently lives in that space. For me, nap time was the first thing to go. I thought that I could come home and take a nap and then start doing my Gerson things, but it hasn't worked out that way. I get home from work, I unpack my Thermos' that hold my juices for work, I drink another juice and I do my coffee enema. Then it is time to start preparing for supper, more supplements and another juice. I prep my green drinks for the morning and have to drink more juice and get ready for another enema before bed. I go to bed at 8:45 so I can get 8 hours. I need to be up by 4:45. Not only did nap time disappear, but watching TV also got crossed off the list pretty fast. I don't go out to dinner for the most part. I don't feel like I have time to go to the movies, which I did a lot. I cancelled my Netflix subscription. Obviously, all my favorite foods are no longer allowed and I also haven't travelled anywhere overnight since I began Gerson therapy. For you, other things might need to go. Hours at the gym, time at Bingo, poker, trivia night, bowling…you will have to fill in the blank. If you are a grandparent, you will absolutely not be able to spend the time with the grandkids that you may be used to. If you have younger children in your home, they may need to learn some new chores to help out and you probably won't be going to any games. I liken doing Gerson therapy to training as an athlete. It takes lots of discipline, lots of resolve, lots of sacrifice and some money too.

What will my doctors think of Gerson Therapy?

Maybe you will have better luck, but my urologists were not supportive of Gerson therapy at all. I asked my first urologist if he had ever heard of Gerson therapy. He said that he had not. When I explained just a little he said that it wouldn't work and I absolutely did not have time to try it. When I asked the 2nd urologist, he just smiled and said, "I don't believe in nutrition therapy." He waved his hand at me as if to say, "enough." He told me of a man who chose a trip to NY for vitamin C IV treatments over chemo. By the time he returned, the cancer had spread and he did not survive. Of course, Gerson therapy is not vitamin C IV treatments. When the second round of medical treatments with Gerson therapy eliminated my cancer, I sent a copy of *Healing the Gerson Way*, with a letter of my good news, to 3 urologists and 2 PCPs. Not one doctor contacted me to acknowledge my gift or congratulate me on my good news. Be prepared for your conventionally trained doctor to be dismissive or even hostile to you opting for Gerson therapy, especially if it means opting not to do chemo or other conventional treatments.

Does Gerson therapy work with medical treatment or all by itself?

Ideally, Gerson therapy works all by itself because, typically, medical treatment will work against the principles that Gerson therapy is founded on. For instance, on Gerson therapy, the patient should not be taking any over the counter or prescription medication. A Gerson trained doctor would need to wean the patient off medications for the therapy to be effective. The reason for this is all medications are toxic. Also, chemotherapy or steroid treatment is also toxic and damaging to the body. If you have been on chemo or other powerful drugs, Gerson therapy may work, but only after your body is able to purge itself of these toxins. In my case, the treatment for bladder cancer is something called BCG. This is in essence, a toxic, but dead, virus placed inside my bladder for a couple hours each week and then evacuated. This virus is supposed to stimulate my immune system. Because the toxin doesn't remain in my body, I have been doing Gerson therapy with the BCG treatments for now. I should be able to stop the BCG treatments and Gerson therapy should be able to heal me all by itself, but I do cheat a little and since the BCG treatment doesn't hurt me as far as I know, I do both as insurance…for now.

I hope this helps. I've tried to give you important information you might need to have if you are in the middle of making decisions. I know from experience, that deciding to forgo a treatment that your doctor is telling you that you NEED to have, in order to do Gerson therapy is a scary proposition. If you choose Gerson therapy, you need to feel like you are choosing of your own volition because you have seen the documentaries or read the book and heard or seen the testimonies and believe that Gerson can and will heal you too! My prayer is that before you subject your body to chemo or other cell damaging drugs, you seriously consider choosing Gerson therapy.

part one

Making the Gerson Therapy Discovery

*Yes, science determines everything, but I often fail
to recognize that God is the scientist.*

I discovered a tumor in my bladder in November. I was diagnosed with bladder cancer, between stage 1 and 2, on December 3rd and I began writing on a website called, Caring Bridge on Dec 16th. When I was diagnosed I decided to be very public about my condition. I honestly felt like if I was talking to anyone, a close friend or just an acquaintance, I wanted to share. Otherwise I felt like I was hiding something. Caring Bridge allowed me to communicate effectively how I was feeling, what happened at the doctor's office, when my next appointment was going to be and what my outlook was. I soon discovered that writing on Caring Bridge was very therapeutic for me and I also felt a connectedness with friends and family that I had not experienced before.

I am not going to share every entry with you, but I am sharing entries that I guess mean the most to me. The purpose of sharing my diary entries with you is so that you can see some of the things you are likely to experience ahead and maybe be prepared for. Also, I want to share things that you can learn from my experience so that you don't have to figure them out on your own. Thirdly, I'm confident that you will benefit from my perspective and positive outlook. Suffering from a life threatening disease can be unnerving, stress inducing and frightening. It may be easy to think like a victim, a victim with no recourse, no power, but to be angry at someone, even yourself, or be depressed or even hopeless. Whether you are a Christian or not, whether you belong to any religious affiliation or not, I have included lots of references to scriptures that have sustained and strengthened me and I think they will strengthen and sustain you as well. Without my Christian experience, meaning, a lifetime of searching out knowledge of God through the Bible and doing my best to apply that knowledge to my life, as well as observing the lives of others striving to do the same, I don't think I would have had the courage or faith to choose Gerson therapy. That same Christian experience teaches me that I should want to share what I have learned with as many people as will listen. When I started writing, I didn't intend to share so much Bible, but every time I set my fingers to the keyboard, scriptures just came to mind, scriptures that fueled my spirit for the challenges I faced.

What you will see in these entries is an intense desire to learn as much as I can and an intense desire to do as much as I possibly can to help my chances for complete healing and recovery. You will see lots of trial and error. You will see me determined to have a good attitude even if I just don't. And I try my best to always measure my cup from the bottom up, not the top down. Let's dive in.

Oh! A note about the book cover: Most books that talk about juicing simply have a glass of delicious looking juice on the book cover. Taking coffee enemas is an integral part of Gerson therapy. I wanted to portray the comfort and peace that I experience during the time I spend in my "Coffee Lounge." Granted, I do a quick water enema before the coffee, making the coffee enema a breeze. This allows me to relax, absolutely, and relish the 15 minutes I spend on my side. Don't be afraid of this. Taking coffee enemas is half the equation to restoring your health.

Marching Forward

December 16, 2012

So, I'm very excited about all that God has been orchestrating for me. Friend Beti has been helping me get fit since July. I've appropriately lost 20 pounds to date. Working out forced me also to radically change my diet and my diagnosis has forced me to change it further. Friend Vivi introduced me to a documentary, *Forks over Knives* and since Nov 24th I've not eaten dairy or meat, including chicken or fish. I'm staying away from refined sugar, flour, table salt and cutting back on oils, yes even olive oil. Surprisingly, this has not been difficult at all. There is plenty of protein in veggies and of course in beans. My new mantra: Food is medicine. Some friends have been seeing energy healer Tom Tam in Quincy. My sister Shelley took me Saturday to a healing session. I felt emotionally great when we left and this session resulted in a very real reduction of pain. Now onto acupuncture, maybe join a Wellness club at the Dedham Whole Foods store. I have felt an amazing wave of love wash over me and hope all that love can be multiplied back in an outward direction…I have another surgery coming up on Dec 26th to finish removing any remaining tumor. Rides are arranged. This is day surgery. Recovery is expected to be a few days. I welcome all the visits I can get at home. YES, that means you have to drive ALL the way to Pembroke. I had great energy after the last surgery and was not bound to my bed. The den is my new hang out. After this surgery, they will give me 4 weeks to heal, then once a week for 6 weeks I will go to the Doc's office. He will insert a synthetic TB into my bladder. I will evacuate the poison after about two hours and this will kick start my body's own antibodies into high gear to attack the TB and any cancer cells left in my bladder. So we will see what happens after that.

Yes, food is my medicine and you are my medicine! Love you, Lynn

Finding my way in Whole Foods

December 17, 2012

Okay, so I made my first serious venture to Whole Foods today. It was a little intimidating. I stood in front of the wall of bins that dispense beans and nuts and seeds and grains. I was trying to figure out, if I dispense into a plastic bag, how will the cashier know what to ring up? How will I even know what I bought? Then I saw, a man was using pint containers and putting labels on the container and then recording a number from the bin onto the label…it's a very precise system.

I was grateful for the flesh and blood example because the stock boy did not give very good instruction. Isn't that the way life so often is. We get all kinds of bad instruction, but sometimes we are lucky enough to run into precious flesh and blood examples that can set us straight if we have the humility to watch and learn. Thank you, all my flesh and blood examples!!

Just a disclaimer: if you usually receive a Christmas card and haven't received a Christmas card from me by now, sorry! I still love you!! I promise :)

The Bible Tells Me So

December 19, 2012

Okay, just thinking out loud. If meat and dairy is so bad for me, why does everyone in the Bible eat meat and dairy? I have a theory. Just because it is in the Bible, doesn't mean it was God's will. After all, everyone in the Bible sinned too. Think about it, do you think there was meat in the Garden of Eden, meat to eat? I don't get the sense that there was. If Adam and Eve had never sinned, they may have been vegans all their lives. Maybe they ate meat in the garden, but I don't think so.

When God instructed Ezekiel to set aside food for 390 days, this is what he said:

Ezekiel 4:9

"Take wheat and barley, beans and lentils, millet and spelt; put them in a storage jar and use them to make bread for yourself. You are to eat it during the 390 days you lie on your side."

When Daniel was taken captive by the Babylonians, he didn't want any part of the rich royal food:

Daniel 1:12-13

"Please test your servants for ten days: Give us nothing but vegetables to eat and water to drink. Then compare our appearance with that of the young men who eat the royal food, and treat your servants in accordance with what you see."

Daniel and his companions seemed healthier after 10 days so they were allowed to continue to eat just veggies. Daniel was in service to 4 different kings and lived into his 80s or maybe older. I'm not sure if he ever added meat back into his diet.

When the Israelites wandered for 40 years in the desert, God provided manna. He gave one meal of quail then 40 years of manna. Exodus 16:11-35

Yes, God instructed the Israelites to eat lamb on the Passover, but it would have been hard to make the parallel to Jesus as the Passover eggplant! God wanted them to be reminded every year that atonement had to be made for their sins.

Yes, God revealed in a vision to Peter that all food was clean, but he was trying to tell Peter that the Gentiles could be saved too!

Paul even says, *Everything is permissible, but not everything is beneficial,* I Corinthians 10:23

I think God provided meat to eat as an alternative when a harvest wasn't readily available. After all, so many people have been nomadic in nature, but I think for the most part we evolved FROM hunters and gatherers TO farmers. I'm open...

No matter, I think the most important scripture about food is Matthew 4:4 *Jesus answered, "It is written: Man does not live on bread alone, but on every word that comes from the mouth of God."*

Not all things are beneficial, but your love is amazingly beneficial to me! Love, Lynn

The Cost of Care

December 20, 2012

I work for a health insurance company so I am always interested in what healthcare costs. Keep in mind, I am otherwise super healthy. I am not on any medications and each year at my physical I always get a clean bill of health. I have had a stress test for my heart, perfect, and all kinds of biometric screenings, A+.

From November 11 to December 11, fourteen insurance claims have been submitted on my behalf totaling, $15,511.32. This includes 4 visits with my urologist and 1 day surgery, also one pre op visit to the hospital. This does not include 2 prescriptions I picked up on the way home from the hospital, the charges of which I don't have ready access to. Let me qualify, this is the total charges. My insurance company is going to pay a far smaller contracted rate.

So when your momma said, "An ounce of prevention is worth a pound of cure," she wasn't kidding. Women usually talk about feelings. I'm a bottom line kind of girl so my feeling is that this dance with cancer is going to wipe out about 5 or 6 years of my investment into the healthcare system and that's the best case scenario. Of course my goal is to always put in more than I take out. This is highly motivating to me. The cost alone of my healthcare is enough to never want to be in this position again. Not to mention the consequences for my actual health or time and energy taken from my normal life schedule. Oh yeah, there are those pesky out of pocket copays and that $1000.00 deductible too; and I have the best insurance money can buy, thankfully.

I tell friends, don't bite off a big mortgage you can barely pay. Give yourself plenty of room and pay it off early. Chances are you will at some point be hit with some hefty medical bills. If you are sick enough to lose your job, you will also lose your insurance. Yikes!

These are just things I happen to chew on, even when I'm healthy.

My goal in my relationship with you? To always put in more than I take out. Love, Lynn!

10 Blessings

December 21, 2012

I awoke at 3:00 this morning and couldn't get back to sleep. I wasn't thinking about me, but just stuff going on with other people, stuff I didn't really want to be thinking about, so I thought it best to start counting, my blessings that is. It's a good way to distract the mind from worry and a good exercise in gratitude:

1. I am more grateful for my Mom, Janet, than I am for anyone else in the world. That's kind of a gimmie, right...her love first of all, her incredible generosity, her shoot from the hip opinions and her amazing, Lucille Ball like, sense of humor.

2. My father, the most gentle man I've ever known, exasperatingly quiet, but who was respected by all and liked by all. He was honest to the core in his dealings, always tipping the scale in favor of others, a man of integrity and worthy of imitation. I especially enjoyed our work together, driving to the dump when I was little, picking out Christmas trees, bringing in the cranberry harvest...any reason to ride in his big pickup truck.

3. My siblings, despite the corporal oppression and abuse in the early years, (I'm the baby)...my sister Shelley, who has been a fabulous example to me in dealing aggressively and assertively with health challenges; my brother Mark who displays almost daily what it means to honor the needs of family above self and my brother Steven who can outwork anyone I know, solely supporting a wife and 4 children by the sweat of his brow since the tender age of 18, his bride just 16 years old.

4. I'm grateful for Pembroke, the town I grew up in. More than anything, this town has offered me quiet spaces in which to ponder all of life's happenings. We had an empty field next to our house growing up. The neighborhood kids used it as their own and no one ever told us not to use it for anything...oh well there was that one time I was shooting my arrows and accidentally put a hole in the neighbors pool lining. The local popo and the neighbor were none too happy. I shot up, aiming for the woods....oops!

5. Camp Four Winds. This was a day camp right in Pembroke that I attended faithfully 8 weeks every summer from the age of 6 to 18. It was 30 beautiful and rustic acres that used to sit on the edge of Hobomock pond. That's where I learned to swim and swim we did! I could probably still tread water for hours. That's where I fell in love with, I know it sounds crazy, folk dancing and eventually became the folk dance instructor, oh yeah...and the archery instructor. Good thing they didn't do a background check with the local police.

6. My first real job at Cataldi's restaurant in Hanson, currently the Meadowbrook. I started clearing tables there at 16 and stayed 6 years. That job paid for my first car, in full, at 17; the down payment for my first house when I was 19; and my college education at Massasoit Community College.

7. My first car, an Oldsmobile Cutlass, a true muscle car, 8 cylinders, 350 engine, great for the passing lane. It lasted 5 years and I haven't loved a car as much since.

8. My Freshman year English teacher at Silver Lake High School, Leslie Sanderson. She was my Jamie Sommers (the bionic woman for those of you who don't remember, who happened to be a school teacher). She was the standard of right, my hero...what I wanted to be when I grew up. She was my compass for 4 years. Be careful. You never know whose compass you might be.

9. My first crush, at camp, on Frankie Morrielli. He was 12 and I was 10. That boy could waltz. I have not credited anyone since with as much innocence, as much purity of character and intent as I gave him. I miss having the ability to look at someone so uncritically.

10. Fyodor Dostoyevsky's, *Crime and Punishment*, which I first read in 9th grade. This book greatly inspired me in my pursuit of God. It made God's supremacy and his sovereignty undeniable and tangible. I often summarize the gist of the book with this scripture: *Do not be deceived: God cannot be mocked. A man reaps what he sows. The one who sows to please his sinful nature, from that nature will reap destruction; the one who sows to please the Spirit, from the Spirit will reap eternal life*, Galatians 6:7-8

Oh, and one more blessing, YOU! Lots of love, Lynn

Blessings 11 - 20

December 23, 2012

I love words and was thinking about some REally REmarkable words that I'm grateful for that all happen to start with RE:

11. Reconciliation, first and foremost with God

12. Repentance, allowing me to be reconciled with God

13. Repair, my body

14. Rest, my body and mind

15. Restore, my health

16. Recovery, after surgery

17. Relief, found in wholeness

18. Renewal, found in a new year

19. Rebirth, forged in our trials

20. And today, reschedule my appointment to see, "Worlds Away." Not a lost opportunity, just a delayed opportunity.

Much love!! Lynn

Preparation Day

December 24, 2012

In the Jewish tradition, there is Preparation Day, which is the Friday before the Sabbath. Because they cannot work on the Sabbath, they have to prepare everything they need on Friday. Today is my preparation day for my surgery since I really can't do any of the work on Christmas Day.

So a girl has got to do what a girl has got to do. I bit the bullet, (wink, wink) and made an appointment for my first professional massage. I went to a new place called *Life Time Massage Therapy* in South Weymouth on rte. 18. Annie was my therapist. I was a little apprehensive, afraid that I would tense up or get ticklish. I'm very ticklish. Anyway, I had something called Asian Bodywork which is work along meridian points or acupoints. An hour is a very long time, but I really want to do all I can to get my body ready for surgery. She worked from the tips of my ears to the pads of my toes. Very relaxing.

Anyway, will be celebrating Christmas Eve the way any good American family does, eating Chinese food....mmmm that will be interesting. How Vegan ARE the Chinese? Wishing you all your shopping DONE, all your gifts WRAPPED, all the food PREPARED and if you are travelling, your gas tank FILLED, but especially your heart filled with the simple joy of Christ and family.

LOTS of LOVE! Lynn

Surgery

December 26, 2012

My Christmas day was enjoyable as it always is. Hope yours was the same. My surgery is today at 2:45. It was nice to have it a little earlier last time. Besides sleep deprivation, fasting is one of my least favorite activities. I feel bad that some of you have said you would fast for me. When push comes to shove, I might take a bullet for you, but fasting is a whole other ball game. Too bad surgery isn't like running the marathon, where you have to pile up on pasta before the event. I'll do fine as long as I don't forget and swallow something down. That is the biggest threat. I just went shopping and plan on cooking a little for the week before my ride arrives. Maybe I'll tape my mouth.

Love, Lynn

My Nutribullet!

December 29, 2012

Yay! My new Nutribullet finally arrived. You've probably seen the infomercials. I have heard twice now that half the food I consume should be raw. It is not easy to eat a lot of raw food. The Nutribullet makes it easy peasy! Yesterday, I had my first smoothie. The recipe book is broken down into different sections:

Digestion, Circulatory, Immune, Nervous, Endocrine, Skeletal, Muscular. There is a section just on cancer under the immune section. Then: foods for detox, for sleep, for healthy aging, for beauty. It's kind of cool.

My first smoothie I had yesterday I made with frozen kale, an apple, strawberries and mixed nuts.

Today I made one with a cucumber, half an orange, strawberries, mixed nuts, pomegranate seeds, Aloe Vera juice and a little grape juice, Oh yeah and a scoop of my super charged green drink powder from *Trader Joe's*. These are not the best tasting things ever, but not bad and easier than preparing and eating a big salad. Plus, no cooking, no butter, no oils, no salad dressing. This is going to make things a lot easier!

Hey stay warm and careful driving!!! Love!!! Lynn

Resolution

December 31, 2012

OH! Here it is, the day I declare my resolutions!!

I guess I should evaluate 2012 first. Hmmm. I had a funny sort of goal last year. It was to repent. Now, for the unchurched (and churched) repentance is not a bad thing or feeling bad, but simply to see things the way God sees them and to live accordingly. The Bible says repentance brings refreshment. It also says God grants repentance, so that is what I asked, "God, please grant me repentance." I feel like he answered in a really big way. I didn't ask for repentance in any specific area, just repentance. Well, as I noted previously, I have a new found view of my body, of exercise and of food, radically different views from just one year ago. That and my newly changed behaviors satisfy my 2012 goal.

The amazing thing is that for the past 15 years or so, the first resolution on my list was to hit my target weight of 125. Every year, I wrote that goal down and every year I missed it. Well, I'm 125 (on the doctor's scale) and the last 10 lbs I didn't even work for. And just to clarify, this weight loss is the result of a change in perspective, not a result of being sick.

The lesson I learned this year and what I found myself practicing is: If I want to reach a goal I need to also willingly and without hesitation or hindrance, embrace the cost. I've spent too many years wasting time arguing with the universe about the cost. If I want the prize, I just have to buck up and pay the price, whether in relationships, in finances, in fitness or health, I just need to buck up and pay the price!

For 2013? I resolve to put into practice the greatest commandment: Love God first with everything and love my neighbor as myself.

I resolve to be cancer free, fit and healthy, no matter what the price.

I resolve to share what I've learned and what I'm learning with as many people as will listen.

And I resolve to be open to receiving new knowledge even if it flies in the face of what I now know to be true.

HAPPY NEW YEAR! Treat your mind and body well! Love, lots of love to you! Lynn

Silence is Golden, Silence is God

January 4, 2013

One of my favorite scriptures in the Bible is Psalm 46:10

Be still, and know that I am God; I will be exalted among the nations, I will be exalted in the earth.

When I go to yoga class, not any time recently, I think about this verse during our last few minutes of meditation. It is not easy to be still, certainly not easy to still the conscious mind. People often say that we can find God in nature, in the mountains and trees and by a running brook. I wholeheartedly believe we connect with God in nature because of the silence we find there. The verse could easily say, "Be quiet and hear the voice of God."

When you think about it, God stills us, does he not? When we have been awake so many hours and are unable to keep our eyes open one minute longer, he says enough, be still, sleep and let me do my work. Our world is suddenly silent, our conscious mind mute. If you have read any of Deepak Chopra, he believes that God resides in each cell in our body, that the mind resides in each cell of our body, certainly not in our brains. And doesn't that make sense? How else would all those involuntary functions be happening? My conscious mind does not even understand how my body works, so I am not directing its functions. Yes, science determines everything, but I often fail to recognize that God is the scientist.

I fully expect that when I treat my body the way God designed, that his great science will ensure healing. Medicine and surgery only treat symptoms. They are stop gap measures. Man's attempt to heal are only a hacking at the leaves, while God is at the root of the tree bringing about real healing. Of course, what about abuse? What damage is permanent? How many bottles of soda are too many? Our bodies are wastelands and sponges for toxins, mostly man made, if not all man made, including prescription drugs and the processed food we consume. Sometimes the damage is too extensive, we lose an organ, we have scar tissue, the body can't heal because we have robbed God of the tools it takes. What are the tools? The food that God grows, peace in our souls, exercise.

I am actively seeking silence in my life. Noise pummels us at every turn. I'm turning off the radio in the car. I'm turning off the radio on the tread mill. (I might have to shoot the family dog, Lola, if she doesn't stop barking incessantly). Quiet does bring peace to the soul, as long as we are not spending our quiet moments worrying. Whether God resides in our mind or not, I know that when I am quiet my mind and body are better able to respond to God's work, the healing, the fixing, the repair, the filing and processing of our thoughts and experiences.

Stayed home today! Not enough quiet to fix the problems today, but I press on, seeking quiet for my mind and my body. Note to self: Buck up little buckaroo! Just a bump in the road, just a bump in the road...

Remember, the voice you listen to most and are most influenced by is your own. Be sure it is worth listening to. Love you! Lynn

Completely Blessed

January 14, 2013

I was riding home from church with my good friend Lori and she was talking about what a good soldier I am being with my cancer. I said, "Can I say something, can I say that I'm actually having FUN? Am I allowed to say that?" Honestly, I feel like I've hit the lottery.

Overnight, every important relationship in my life got a little deeper, got a little more expressive and got a lot more deliberate. I am freer to express my love. I'm freer to receive love from others. I'm taking tons more time to do both. I am way more focused on people and not as much on tasks. I'm thinking more about what is going on with others and I'm more concerned with what is going on with others.

I guess potentially deadly disease provides a looking glass that brings clarity and focus to the blessings that have been in plain sight, but that have been covered in a veil of familiarity and routine. My family is like solid rock beneath my feet, old faithful friends like a cottage retreat not visited nearly enough, steady friends like safe and favored paths I walk each day and new friends like a cool, bubbling spring of refreshing water. God is like the warmth and light of the sun above that drenches it all. I am completely blessed.

Love you more and more! Lynn

Top Reads for Me

January 15, 2013

I have a little table next to my chair in my den. My large print Bible sits there among the 3 remote controls it takes to watch TV. But lately, it has been getting really crowded on that little table. I have a book on prayer there and two recently purchased books on Tong Ren, the healing methodology I have recently engaged in. Now, those books are buried because I have 4 more recent arrivals and 1 on the way.

Beating Cancer: 20 natural, spiritual, and medical remedies, by Francisco Contreras MD

Eat to Live, by Joel Fuhrman MD

Toxic Relief, by Don Colbert MD

Super Foods: food and medicine of the future, by David Wolfe

Anti-Cancer: A New Way of Life, by David Servan-Schreiber MD

Read well, read often!! Love you, Lynn

Precious Stones

January 21, 2013

What makes a stone precious? It's rarity? Yes, its rarity. I don't believe I own any "Precious Stones." I don't think I ever have. I do not desire to own them for the sake of owning them.

Yet, I do possess stones of great value. A friend recently gave me a small bag with 3 "healing" stones in it. One is called Bloodstone, also called, "The Hero's Stone." It is said that Medieval Christians often used bloodstone to carve scenes of the crucifixion and martyrs, leading it to also be dubbed "Martyr's stone."

These are precious to me because of the giver, someone who had me on her heart, someone concerned about my healing and who wanted to convey that concern. I carry that polished green and crimson bloodstone in my pocket almost every day to remind me of the giving and of the giver.

It is said of Jesus:

Acts 4:11

Jesus is 'the stone you builders rejected, which has become the cornerstone.'

Romans 9:33

As it is written: "See, I lay in Zion a stone that causes people to stumble and a rock that makes them fall, and the one who believes in him will never be put to shame."

1 Peter 2:3-6

"As you come to him, the living Stone—rejected by humans but chosen by God and precious to him— you also, like living stones, are being built into a spiritual house to be a holy priesthood, offering spiritual sacrifices acceptable to God through Jesus Christ. For in Scripture it says:

"See, I lay a stone in Zion,
a chosen and precious cornerstone,

*and the one who trusts in him
will never be put to shame."*

Jesus is a rare stone indeed; the most precious. Value is bestowed on him only because of the giver. That giver has given this stone to me and you.

Ecclesiastes 3:5 says that there is a time to gather stones and a time to scatter them. Gather your precious stones.

As my friend Steve would say, "More love, more love," Lynn

Xs and Os

January 24, 2013

Do you remember the first time someone signed a card to you with "XO"? I do not. Maybe it was when I was a kid in summer camp and I wrote to friends over the winter, kids who lived really far away like in Canton :) The Xs and Os made the letters special of course. Now in this world of virtual relationships, I find the Xs and Os all the more relevant. Hey, I started texting only in the last couple years so the novelty has not worn off. And now I have been working from home so that means more and more emails and text messages.

When I was in college and sharing a big beautiful house with friends in RI, my pillow case, that zips onto the pillow, tore. One of my housemates sewed up the tear and when she gave it back to me I saw that she had stitched in XOX. It warmed my heart. Yesterday, I was talking on Facebook to a friend in CA. He sent me XO 2 or 3 times in the same conversation. It warmed my heart. I sent an XO to a friend yesterday and she sent back XOXOXO. It warmed my heart. And isn't it kind of special, when a relationship with an acquaintance takes a turn and you receive that first XO? Almost gives me goose bumps.

"X" marks the kiss on the wings of angels from me to you and "O" marks a hug around the neck and a bushel and a peck of love.

And God too sends me an XO; the X that is the cross, on which Jesus hanged and the O that was his thorny crown.

(Just an aside... I'm tempted to think maybe I'm giving you too much Jesus for your palate's taste, but I would ask that you consider what God might think of that opinion....Jesus himself said, "If they keep quiet, the stones will cry out.")

XOXOXO, Lynn

Yoga, a Together Experience

January 30, 2013

I had never been interested in the least, in "practicing" yoga. Up until a couple years ago, many friends had suggested it or invited me along and I conveniently discovered a reason I could not go, like, "I don't wanna." That changed about 2 years ago, when an acquaintance invited me. I knew it was a way for me to spend time with someone I wanted to get to know so I bit the bullet and went. The class was hot power yoga. It is about 95 degrees in the class. The first few times I thought I was going to faint. I'm glad I went! Now I have a solid friendship, a fantastic yoga instructor and all the benefits of hot power yoga.

The yoga instructor always emphasizes that we are not to be trying to do what our neighbor is doing, that my experience is between me and my body and me and my mat. But that is just not the way it goes for me. Having a friend by my side is half the experience. My ears and eyes are on my instructor, but my peripheral vision is always informing me of my friend's movement, her ease or her difficulty, her breathing. There isn't competition on a yoga mat, but rather an indirect and silent, but powerful companionship, a partnership, at least for me. I liken it to two friends rock climbing. Can I extend my legs like that? Can I breathe into my twist like that? Her strength and her flexibility inspire me to explore my own limits just a little more. You model for one another, you inspire one another and when a move is ridiculously difficult you exchange a glance with raised eyebrows or a giggle. I really like the congruent movement. We are like synchronized swimmers and I feel like our souls are somewhat synchronized as well.

A friend told me last week that each one of us has an energy field and that energy field can extend outwards up to 15 feet. Since that first visit to yoga, I have enjoyed yoga with a few good friends and I revel in the shade of that good energy, in the bathing of that good energy. There is no talking in yoga. It is just a quiet place of peace and a simple understanding that for a time, we are together.

Namaste, (my soul greets your soul), with love, Lynn

Healing Soup

January 31, 2013

After my first surgery, my friend Steve came by the house with soup from Whole Foods and Au Bon Pain. He was paying attention to my diet and knew what to give me for healing. One day I stopped by the Cedar Cafe restaurant in Hanover to chat with that fabulous Greek family who owns the place. They convinced me to have a little lunch and though I didn't ask, matriarch Nopy came from behind the counter with a large bowl of her spectacular soup for me. She knew my diet and assured me that everything in there was just what I needed for healing. Monday was my last day at work. Coworker Colleen knows of my diet and gave me a big container of healing soup. Cousin Lisa sat in my kitchen on Tuesday night with a large bowl of hot mushroom and onion soup. Just what the good Dr. Fuhrman ordered for my healing.

Isn't it grand when friends and family know us well enough to give us exactly what we need for healing!! Ideally the body wants to be in a state of homeostasis, a state in which the body's internal environment is kept stable. And that is what healing is all about.

God also knows exactly what we need for spiritual homeostasis. His office visit consists of repentance and forgiveness and then he prescribes this soup for health maintenance. He starts with a broth of faith and then adds a list of his own special ingredients:

2 Peter 1:3-8

His divine power has given us everything we need for a godly life through our knowledge of him who called us by his own glory and goodness...For this very reason, make every effort to add to your faith goodness; and to goodness, knowledge; and to knowledge, self-control; and to self-control, perseverance; and to perseverance, godliness; and to godliness, mutual affection; and to mutual affection, love. For if you possess these qualities [ingredients] in increasing measure, they will keep you from being ineffective and unproductive in your knowledge of our Lord Jesus Christ.

Love, Lynn

Gleaning

February 1, 2013

Gleaning is the act of collecting leftover crops from farmers' fields after they have been harvested. From the time I was 6 to about 17, my folks owned a cranberry bog in Hanson. We all weeded and we all harvested, everyone with his or her own job. I always knew that there was a lot of crop left behind after we dry picked. We could not afford to wet pick. The especially big beautiful berries grew on the edges of the ditches where no machine could get to. And it always really bothered me that we were leaving all those berries to rot on the vine. I probably would have done more to get those berries except for the fact that I don't like cranberries and had I actually found a way to pick them, I didn't really have anyone I could give them to. The birds did all the gleaning.

Now, I am into a different kind of gleaning. Of late, I have been in a serious learning mode because of my cancer diagnosis, learning from books and videos (my favorite way). However, in July I got serious about working out and most everything I learned was from a friend who just happens to love to work out. It was scheduled and deliberate learning. That was sort of like harvesting in a field untouched, rich with plenty of crop.

I've also made a habit of when I travel, to see what I can glean on the trip, either from the habits and culture of the environment or something from my host or hostess. This is more subtle, more like gleaning from a harvested field. My learning is still deliberate, but happenstance, unscheduled and random.

Now, more and more, I find myself making a point to glean in all my relationships. What does this person have in their field, their orchard or their garden of habits, traits, qualities or knowledge that I can learn and apply to my own life? This act of gleaning makes my relationships richer. I am more consciously appreciating all the tremendous facets of a friend's being, who they are, their rich and unique experiences, their strengths and gifts.

Do we stop being students after we get our degree? Is the only place we learn new things on the job? Are the only people we learn from those with titles? God forbid! However, gleaning requires that you start from a position of humility. And true humility requires a true sense of security. You have to know your own value to practice humility. A prideful man cannot learn from others easily because he will not bow down to reap.

Happy harvesting! Love, Lynn

As a Man Thinketh

February 2, 2013

Can I share some words from one of my very favorite books of all time? *As a Man Thinketh* was written by James Allen sometime between 1902 and 1912. It is a challenging book because of the English used to write it. And yet, the language and concepts within are beautiful and compelling. I have looked and

I cannot find in the Bible, "As a man thinks, so he is." I thought for sure it was in the book of Proverbs, but it is eluding me. Anyway, Allen says:

'As a man thinketh in his heart so is he,' not only embraces the whole of man's being, but is so comprehensive as to reach out to the very condition and circumstance of his life. A man is literally what he thinks, his character being the complete sum of all his thoughts.

As the plant springs from, and could not be without, the seed, so every act of a man springs from the hidden seeds of thought, and could not have appeared without them....

Just as a gardener cultivates his plot, keeping it free from weeds, and growing the flowers and fruits which he requires, so may a man tend the garden of his mind, weeding out all the wrong, useless, and impure thoughts, and cultivating toward perfection the flowers and fruit of right, useful and pure thoughts. By pursuing this process, a man sooner or later discovers that he is the master-gardener of his soul, the director of his life. He also reveals, within himself, the laws of thought, and understands, with ever increasing accuracy, how the thought-forces and mind elements operate in the shaping of his character, circumstances and destiny.

I have been thinking about this a lot. People ask me how I am doing emotionally. If I had been struck with cancer at 25, I'm not sure how I would be doing, but at 51 I have been cultivating my garden a long time and deliberately so. I remember that at only 20 I was extremely critical, skeptical and negative. I did not have a favorable view of many people or much in the world. I was mostly not happy and far from joyful. I was cautious and untrusting and mostly kept to myself.

I also realized at some point that I did not like being any of those things and the only way to change was from the inside out. The more I read and the more I watched others, the more I realized the power of my own internal voice and how the words and thoughts I allowed or did not allow in my head could and most absolutely would mold my view of myself and the world around me. As my perspective changed so I changed and my life changed.

Why would I want to remain in the former way of thinking when I could be and have something different? Life is way too short. Why would I waste one more minute in a place I don't want to be in? A change in thinking and in perspective takes time, maybe years of correcting all the familiar pathways in the brain, but deciding to change only takes a second. What are you waiting for?

The scripture I DID find is 2 Corinthians 10:5 *We take captive every thought to make it obedient* to Christ. God is telling us we have the power to change our thoughts and thus ourselves. Oh, so how am I doing? It only took me 51 years to get here, but never better in my life. Thanks for asking.

Love you!!!! (at least that's what I keep telling myself), Lynn

One Right Choice 1000 Times

February 8, 2013

I was having a conversation with a friend who knows he needs to deal with his health by changing his diet, but he is just unwilling to make the change. I try to use logic to appeal and persuade, but no luck. He says, "I believe, I believe." But he doesn't really. Joel Fuhrman would say he is a philosophical dieter where as I am a practicing dieter. So what is the problem?? He believes in the concept but does not want to accept the details.

"I know I should lose weight, but this bag of chips isn't going to make a difference." The reality is that one bag won't make a difference, but making the right choice 1000 times will. Unfortunately, making one bad choice 1000 times will also.

"I know I should spend time with my kids, but time together doesn't seem to make a difference in their attitude." How about spending time with your kids 1000 times? How about dinner together 1000 times?

"I know I should get my debt under control, but its thousands of dollars, what's one more pair of shoes?" The reality is it has been lots of shoes, clothes and jewelry you can do without; Starbucks, dinner out, Amazon and on and on. Instead of adding $50.00 to the bill each month, how about paying the interest plus $50.00 each month? And then do that 1000 times.

What we believe in is excuses. What we believe in is comfort. What we believe in is "easy." What we believe in is "later." We don't know what self-control even feels like. We don't understand or experience delayed gratification. We can't comprehend the idea of taking one step at a time, one day at a time, one week at a time. "Persistence" is not in our vocabulary. "Resolve" is not in our vocabulary. "I will, no matter the cost," is not in our vocabulary.

How many times must a 12 year old boy throw a lasso before reigning in a calf? And then how many times must he throw a lasso before he can rein in that little calf while riding a horse. How many times do you think? 1000 times? I have no idea. But whether it is 100 or 10,000, he will learn. He will do it, because he has decided to do it.

Our bad habits are like little calves just waiting to be reined in, but if you are not willing to pick up the rope, if you are not willing to practice and practice and practice a thousand times; that little calf may as well be a greased pig. You see the little calf as a greased pig and as impossible, simply impossible, to catch. And you tell yourself, "I'm not diving into the muck to catch that little greased piggy."

Come on, man!

Put some walk into your talk.

Put some do into your belief.

Put some practice into your preaching.

You can't learn how to swim unless you get in the water. You can't rein in those bad habits if you are unwilling to train with the right tools 1000 times over.

So here you go. You have 3 days in a lab, a closed system: Friday, Saturday and Sunday, with the assistance of storm Nemo. What did Jonah learn in 3 days? What did Paul learn in 3 days when knocked to the ground? God seems to be saying 3 days is a good incubation period. You can kick start your 1000 choices in 3 days!

Stop groveling. Stand up! Rise up! Ready! Set! Go!

Yeah, I believe...in you!!!! Love, Lynn

A Needed Love Letter

February 14, 2013

A love letter from Hosea today.

Hosea 2:14-20

Therefore I am now going to allure her;
I will lead her into the desert
and speak tenderly to her.
There I will give her back her vineyards,
and will make the Valley of Achor a door of hope.
There she will sing as in the days of her youth,
as in the day she came up out of Egypt.
"In that day," declares the Lord,
"you will call me 'my husband';
you will no longer call me 'my master'...
I will betroth you to me forever;
I will betroth you in righteousness and justice,
in love and compassion.
I will betroth you in faithfulness,
and you will acknowledge the Lord.

David was a man familiar with challenges so I inquired of him:

Psalm 108:1-6

My heart is steadfast, O God;
I will sing and make music with all my soul.
Awake, harp and lyre!
I will awaken the dawn.
I will praise you, O Lord, among the nations;
I will sing of you among the peoples.
For great is your love, higher than the heavens;
your faithfulness reaches to the skies.

Be exalted, O God, above the heavens,
and let your glory be over all the earth.
Save us and help us with your right hand,
that those you love may be delivered.

On this Valentine's Day, loving you! Lynn

A Patient's View

February 17, 2013

I started reading my second cancer book, *Anti Cancer: A New Way of Life* by David Servan-Schreiber, MD, PhD. He is a doctor who found himself with a cancerous brain tumor. He is very articulate. I want to share some of his words.

When we put off till tomorrow the quest for the essential, we may find life slipping through our fingers without ever having savored it. Cancer sometimes cures this strange nearsightedness, this dance of hesitations. By exposing life's brevity, a diagnosis of cancer can restore life's true flavor. A few weeks after my diagnosis, I had the odd feeling a veil had been lifted that until then had dimmed my sight. One Sunday afternoon...I was looking at Anna [his girlfriend]...For the first time, I saw her as she was...I simply saw the lock of hair that slipped gracefully forward when she leaned her head on her book, the delicacy of her fingers gently grasping the pen. I was surprised that I had never noticed how touching the slightest contractions of her jaw could be when she had trouble finding the word she was looking for...Her presence became incredibly moving. Simply being allowed to witness that moment came to me as an immense privilege...Thus, the approach of death can sometimes lead to a kind of liberation. In its shadow, life suddenly takes on an immensity, resonance, and savor we may never have known before.

I felt this in the first few days of my diagnosis, not that I think, at this point, I am going to die of this diagnosis. It is very hard to describe, but the grays of life take on vibrant color. It is a little like falling in love. Everything is beautiful. Everything is wondrous. Every moment is to be absorbed through all the senses at their height and what cannot be taken in through the senses, I pray to absorb through the pores of my skin.

He goes on to say, *Gentle, constant, reliable presence is often the most beautiful gift our dear ones can give us.*

I find this to be absolutely true... Thank you for your presence!!! Without it, there would be little meaning, if any at all.

PRESENTLY thinking of you, love, Lynn

Novel Idea

February 18, 2013

Everything I am learning about cancer and disease in general suggests that in addition to receiving traditional western medical treatment, a patient can and should be taking a greater role of responsibility by adding these five habits:

1) Detoxification of carcinogenic substances and pollutants

2) An anti-cancer diet, which means whole foods, plant based, and a little, if any, grass fed red meat or chicken and a small amount, if any, of small fish like sardines. The reason for limiting fish is toxins and pollutants in the water, no dairy

3) Regular exercise, 30 minutes, 6 times a week

4) Emotional peace through stress reduction, which could include more and better quality sleep, meditation or other forms of stress reduction

5) Emotional support by building, engaged, expressive personal relationships

So, if this is what is good for someone with serious illness, my guess is that this is good for someone who does not have serious illness, yet. Stats show that rates of cancer, heart disease and diabetes are all way up. In addition, disease is showing up in younger and younger patients. And to top it off, modern western medicine does not supply any cures, but only serves as crisis management, addressing the symptoms of disease. Why do you think they are called "Maintenance drugs?" Again, as I mentioned before, western medicine is a hacking at the leaves. My sister said to me, "once a cancer patient, always a cancer patient." My doctor implied as much. My father had serious melanoma at the age of 70. After radical surgery and treatments, he was in remission for 10 years. Then the cancer came back with a vengeance from the inside out. Only our bodies can cure cancer and other disease. That's why the 5 habits above are critical to a long, healthy life. Please don't depend on your doctor to "heal" you. He does not have that power. Even the treatments I will receive in the doctor's office depend on my immune system to do the work. That is why bladder cancer is one of the least threatening cancers.

I'm reminded of that old commercial. "One of these days you are going to break down and call me." I think it was for Triple A. Sooner or later, you will break down and call your doctor. After you hang up with her, call me!

Scared straight, Lynn, with love, Lynn

Perseverance

February 23, 2013

Perseverance: *steady persistence in a course of action, a purpose, a state, etc., especially in spite of difficulties, obstacles, or discouragement.*

Yesterday at yoga, the instructor Emma called upon my friend to demonstrate a pose that no one else in the class has mastered yet, a Pincha Mayurasana or forearm stand. You start with your forearms on the floor and your feet squarely behind you and you work your way into a forearm stand, your head never touching the floor. To say it takes incredible strength and balance is an understatement. Emma noted that it took hours upon hours of practice to achieve this skill level. My friend whispered twice that she had practiced so much her arms bled, not unlike many determined athletes.

This made me think of two scriptures that I had no idea were just 3 verses away from each other. We are all persevering in one struggle or another and whether we like it or not we are all running a race to an eternal end. Hebrews chapter 11 is called the, *Hall of Fame of Faith* because it recounts the stories of many great men and women of faith and the hardships they faced to finish their lives faithful to God, many shedding their blood to do so. In view of their incredible examples, chapter 12 begins, "Therefore...

Hebrews 12:1

Therefore, since we are surrounded by such a great cloud of witnesses, let us throw off everything that hinders and the sin that so easily entangles, and let us run with perseverance the race marked out for us.

Then he talks about Jesus and his perseverance, even to death on the cross, shedding his blood for us.

Hebrews 12:4

In your struggle against sin, you have not yet resisted to the point of shedding your blood.

Isn't it funny that we probably think it fanatical that someone might shed their blood for a goal, but if Jesus hadn't for us, we would have no doorway to heaven. But now, the writer of Hebrews also warns, look, Jesus did his part, now you have to do your part. Don't be surprised if it takes a little blood, sweat and tears.

You and me, persevering in our love and life. Love, Lynn

Building...

March 4, 2013

Having this cancer diagnosis is sort of like getting a new dog, a puppy, untrained, with lots of energy and demanding lots of attention. I know this is not the case with many people who get a cancer diag. I think there are many who keep it close to the chest, go to work, go to treatments and try to keep life as normal as possible.

I, on the other hand, have fully embraced this moment to take quantum leaps in my learning. Actually, I don't even feel it is a choice. I feel absolutely compelled. My appetite for books and videos is insatiable and my desire to share is equal in strength. In many ways I feel betrayed, by Western Medicine first and foremost, by my doctor whose indifference delayed my diagnosis, by the food industry who sells us junk, by the government that promotes and sustains big agribusiness and ranching that is destroying our earth and our bodies and uses tax subsidies to do it, etc.

I feel like I am very much in a building phase. I'm building knowledge, building new habits, new values and building my resources to share with others. Our little group that meets Friday nights is good. We continue to learn and put into practice the info we are gaining. I am building a personal library - I bought 7 new books today!! And I'm building a list of helpful videos. Let me share a few today that deal specifically with cancer. I have not seen any of these but am confident the message is aligned with my values (just by the titles). A special thanks to all those who send me tips and leads...

Dying to have Known (About Gerson Therapy)

Beautiful Truth (About Gerson Therapy)

The Gerson Miracle (About Gerson Therapy)

Happy Viewing! Love, Lynn

Max Gerson

March 5, 2013

I watched 2 of the videos I mentioned yesterday. They were about Gerson therapy based on the work of Max Gerson and his treatment, without drugs, of his cancer patients. Since no double blind studies can be performed to "prove" his therapy as scientifically sound he was banned from US medical journals and dismissed by the medical community in the 50s. However,

Gerson therapy hospitals in Mexico and Japan are thriving with more on the way. There were plenty of patients on hand to testify to their cures, patients who had been given a death sentence by their own doctors. Max Gerson died of arsenic at the age of 86.

Max Gerson's work preceded the ground breaking studies of

T. Colin Campbell PhD and Caldwell Esselstyn MD on the dangers of dairy and animal products, which preceded books by

Dean Ornish MD and John Robbins MD on the benefits of a vegetarian diet.

Joel Fuhrman MD and David Servan- Schrieber MD stand on the shoulders of all these giants in their prescription of diet along with medical treatment for the reversal and cure of most disease including cancer, heart disease and diabetes.

Believe it or not! Love, Lynn

The Gerson Miracle

March 6, 2013

So I just have to tell you, I watched, *The Gerson Miracle* last night on Netflix. It is by far the most informative on Max Gerson and his amazing cancer treatment. However, of all the info and all the patient testimony, I think the most amazing is Charlotte Gerson talking about her own health. She is almost 90, probably has never taken a drug in her life, still working and fit as a fiddle. If anyone feels they may be failing in their personal fight against cancer, I'm betting that Gerson therapy is the way to go.

Lots of love and health to you, Lynn

Candle Light!

March 15, 2013

During the Christmas season, my mom asked me if I had noticed the candle light in the neighbors' window. There was a single candle facing my house that was lit for me in vigil as I faced my cancer journey. After Christmas season was over and all the houses in the neighborhood went dark, that candle still stood in its place. My neighbors went away for some time on vacation. They recently returned and wouldn't you know it, the candle is lit again and in the window. I know the Mrs. stays in touch with my mom and asks about how I am doing. I almost feel bad that it is still lit. I don't know how long they will keep it up.

When I see that candle I am reminded of a prophecy about Jesus.

Isaiah 42:3

A bruised reed he will not break, and a smoldering wick he will not snuff out.

How often can we feel like a bruised reed or feel like we are just squeaking by, barely making it day to day? This verse says Jesus sees and he is there to help, not harm, to support, not crush. He can nurture a bruised reed and fan into flame a smoldering wick. Literally when he breathes into us, he inspires us. He is gently blowing on the embers, glowing!

Lots of love to you! Lynn

Epidemic?

March 24, 2013

An epidemic occurs when new cases of a certain disease, in a given human population, and during a given period, substantially exceed what is expected based on recent experience.

When I was growing up, the stat always thrown around was 1 in 4. One in four people would get cancer in their lifetime. Now the rates are way up. The National Cancer Institute now says, "Based on rates from 2007-2009, 41.24% of men and women born today will be diagnosed with cancer at some time during their lifetime. This number can also be expressed as 1 in 2 men and women will be diagnosed with cancer of all sites during their lifetime." When I say I have cancer or I quote this alarming rate, the response of most is, "Well, they can do so much more for cancer today than they could even just a few years ago." That understood, why would we still not be trying to figure out the cause and do something to prevent getting cancer? Well, because if you are like me, you simply think, it will be someone else. Unfortunately, once I got my diagnosis, I'm kind of stuck with this ongoing treatment. It's VERY costly on many levels.

In the early 1900s cancer was extremely rare. And as we see cancer rates increase all over the globe, the only thing that coincides with that increase is the spread of the Standard American Diet. In the early 80s I feared that the spread of AIDS would be the downfall of our health care system. On the horizon, it seems that diabetes and obesity may be the downfall of our health care system, but right up there is heart disease and cancer rates that have exploded in the last few decades. These current rates of disease in society are not sustainable. We blame health care costs for squeezing our budgets at every level. Health care costs are the symptom. Poor health is the problem. Our poor health is directly linked to our increased consumption of animal products, highly processed foods and toxins in our food sources and environment. Oh yeah, and that we are consuming on average 30% more calories than we need on any given day. I encourage you, as my friend always says, do your homework. Figure it out, don't wait for the diagnosis. Many, if not most people think cancer is random and just strikes haphazardly. If you believe you have no power, then you will have no power. Yes, perhaps the sky IS falling.

Find your power! Lot of love! Lynn

My Declaration

April 5, 2013

I was talking about my upcoming biopsy surgery that is happening on Tuesday and my empathetic listener said something about going through the "Horror" of having cancer. I had to say once again that, horror is not anything I have come close to experiencing and in fact I have experienced the EXACT opposite. I told her, I have received so much love that I have no choice but to be the happiest I've ever been in my life. And it's not something I have to work at with my head. My heart is full. I feel the incredible support of my incredible family and friends and I feel close to God. I don't feel cursed. I feel blessed. I also mistakenly said that I deal with cancer with prayer. That was too short an answer. I deal with cancer with 35 years of prayer under my belt, Bible study and faith building relationships.

I feel like this is just God telling me loudly and clearly, "Lynn, you have not been making right choices and you need to make different ones. Let me help you understand so that you can be as I designed you to be." I can't make sense of everyone's cancer. I can only hope to learn and heal and grow from my own cancer. My declaration is this: If I live, amen. If I perish, I perish, (favorite words from the book of Esther). Either way, it is well with my soul.

Psalm 40:5

Many, Lord my God, are the wonders you have done, the things you planned for us. None can compare with you; were I to speak and tell of your deeds, they would be too many to declare.

Declaring my love for you! Lynn

Sinking Ice

April 9, 2013

Biopsy surgery today showed more tumor growth in my bladder. I will meet with the doc on Tues to evaluate plans going forward

Keep praying and thank you!

Love, Lynn

One Day at a Time

April 11, 2013

One of the toughest parts of being sick is trying to plan for anything at all. The difficulty of this surgery caught me off guard. I guess because it was called "biopsy surgery" I thought it was going to be quick and easy. So now, how much work do I need to take off? I can't say when I will return. I know it is challenging for folks at work because I have also waited for people to return to work. I know what it feels like. It is also difficult to say that I can work or cannot work from home.

I am taking my new drug and am staying away from the pain killers. The new drug is working to minimize spasms, but not completely. I think my body prefers me lying down. It seems I can go some length also sitting, but standing and walking around seems to trigger the spasms. I am making sure I eat well. I didn't eat so much after the last two surgeries, but I want to make a concerted effort to get the maximum amount of nutrition. I guess, one day at a time.

I was hoping to see the doctor by Tuesday afternoon, but got bumped to Wednesday. Not sure how long to keep this catheter in. Seven days seems like a long time. Yikes!

Proverbs 19:21

Many are the plans in a person's heart, but it is the Lord's purpose that prevails.

Planning on loving you always! Lynn

Cross Roads

April 12, 2013

My head is a little all over. A little anxious about what my options are going forward. I hadn't really planned on this first round of BCG not completely eradicating all cancer cells. I've decided to put off my trip to Greece. I don't want to try to do too much just for the sake of doing it. I was looking today more intently at different treatment centers that practice Gerson therapy. These are facilities that use nutrition and detox, only, to reverse and heal cancer and other disease. The original Gerson hospital is in Mexico. There are at least two more like it in Mexico. I looked at one in Sedona, very ritzy and one in California. The idea is I would go and stay for 10 to 14 days and learn how to do the program while I am there and then continue when I return home. I don't exactly know how long I would need to continue the regimen at home. It's pretty intense. All the facilities do it the exact same way. 13 glasses of freshly juiced fruits and veggies and coffee enemas during the day to keep the liver safe while it detoxes all the junk out of your body. Yes, that is the least appealing, almost off putting part of the program. The program works best if the patient hasn't had chemo or radiation. I'll poke around to see if I can find anything on the east coast. Of course insurance does not pay. This would be why I save for a rainy day. It's raining.

The theory behind this is the same I've seen in everything I've read and watched. The body will heal itself if given the right tools. This Gerson therapy is like Joel Fuhrman's diet or the *Forks over Knives* diet intensified. Of course I need to wait and see what the doc says, but I haven't been having any fun at all doing this the traditional way and not getting the results I want either. We'll see. Pray for God to guide me.

James 1:5

If any of you lacks wisdom, you should ask God, who gives generously to all without finding fault, and it will be given to you.

He gave me the wisdom to love you! Lynn

On the Offense

April 13, 2013

For 4 days since my surgery I had pretty much been in a defeated mode, hijacked, if you will, by anesthesia and scalpels and drugs and devices and pain. Today, a new strategy. Today I'm ramping up my game. I've been really good about eating lots of veggies and fruit, beans, nuts and seeds. I have not been super vigilant about making sure it is all organic. Today, I bought all organic and I finally got around to switching out all my toiletries. I got Tom's fluoride free toothpaste and aluminum free deodorant. I bought organic shampoo, conditioner, body wash and moisturizer.

I was giving more thought to and reading more about Gerson therapy and I think it may not be a good fit. Practicing the therapy is a full time job literally and the treatment at home could last as much as 9 months to more than 2 years depending on my body's response. Hmmm… now thinking, maybe I just want to join Dr. Fuhrman's "member center" and get more tied in there.

What was that scripture? Oh yeah...

James 1:2-4

Consider it pure joy, my brothers and sisters, whenever you face trials of many kinds, because you know that the testing of your faith produces perseverance. Let perseverance finish its work so that you may be mature and complete, not lacking anything.

My joy is complete when I consider you. Love, Lynn

My Brain is Tired

April 14, 2013

Since the discovery in November of my tumor in my bladder, my brain has just been going and going trying to figure out the solution to this cancer problem. I think it is just a normal survival instinct and compulsion. During my BCG treatment, my brain got a rest because I was on track, doing what I needed to do to handle the problem. Since the discovery of more tumor growth on Tuesday, my brain has been reactivated and now is just tired of trying to find the answer. I have to just take the night off, escape into a movie or something. The more I read the more complicated it gets and the more questions I have about how my body really works, how it really interacts with the environment and with food. Yeesh!

My new doctor says bladder cancer happens because of exposure to chemicals. Was it all the spraying on the cranberry bogs I live near or on the bogs we owned and worked on? Something else? Smokers have a higher incidence of bladder cancer than non-smokers. Was it working in that smoke filled restaurant for six years? Was it the smoke in my home, growing up? The questions come. The "How" questions don't even matter, but the "What now?" questions are challenging to quiet.

I'm glad my great hope is not in this life, but there are precious many I love here. Love, Lynn

Mourning with Marathoners

April 15, 2013

I think about how hard I am working to improve my health, the hours, the months, the planning, all the calculating, the work just for small improvements and then I think of innocent people, healthy and strong, in an instant losing everything, even life itself. And I think of the dozens of others whose bodies and souls will never be the same, lost limbs, terrible wounds, forever scarred by pure evil, always feeling loss… always feeling loss. THAT would challenge me to the core. No accident, no negligence, but deliberate, directed evil.

God have mercy! Sending love, even in chaos, Lynn

Tough Day

April 17, 2013

My fear was that my doc would say that he needs to take my bladder out. Today that fear was realized. He said if the BCG treatment doesn't work, then that's it. There is no other viable treatment left. Chemo doesn't work and radiation doesn't work and if BCG didn't work the first time, it won't work the second time. He says my immune system is shot and the tissue of my bladder looks like that of an 80 year old. The people who get bladder cancer are old men who have smoked for decades. I'm not even a candidate for bladder cancer, never mind cancer that does not respond to treatment. I actually brought up Gerson therapy and naturally he had never heard of it and dismissed it immediately. Again, rethinking. Will be on the phone with Gerson Hospital tomorrow to find out what kind of history they have with high grade, aggressive bladder cancer where the recommendation is to remove the bladder.

I REALLY, REALLY appreciate all the support, the comments and the prayers. I so thought this was going to be a piece of cake. Please pray for healing, and also that God makes my path REALLY, REALLY clear.

Lots of love, from me to you! Lynn

part two

Turning to Gerson in Desperation

*I'm fighting to hold the line. I'm pushing hard to
gain a hair line, a fraction of a millimeter.*

On April 17th, 2012, my urologist told me that my medical treatment failed completely and that I would have to have my bladder removed within two weeks because this aggressive, high grade cancer would surely spread quickly through the wall of my bladder and spread throughout the rest of my body. Just a week and a half earlier, I was winding down my treatment mindset. I was already making plans for work and my home and other projects I wanted to start. I was grateful all this cancer stuff was coming to an end, confident that the BCG treatments would completely eradicate my bladder cancer. My head was now spinning.

I tried with all my heart to ensure that I was doing everything I could to vanquish this enemy within. When my efforts failed, I was crushed, of course. Receiving such scary news is like being in a nightmare. I kept thinking, "How can this be possible?" This radical surgery that my doctor was insisting I needed was certainly not in my plan. I kept trying to envision what life would be like without a bladder. I hate, really hate, having any kind of physical malady, short term or long. My brain would not accept the fact that I would have no way of fixing, "no badder." Once it is taken out, that's it!! There is no getting it back. Then there would be a lifetime of maintenance, probably complications and lots more medical treatment. I kept trying to picture doing yoga with a bag attached. On top of all that, the doctor admitted that the survival rate of people who have their bladders out is only 50% after 5 years. What? Nope, this could not be. In a crisis, I always go to the positive stance first. I was wavering, but I kept saying to myself, "There has got to be a better way." I kept coming back to Gerson therapy.

In the pages to come, you will see me dig in, reset my mind and my spirit to find an acceptable solution and all the decisions I had to make to get to that solution.

I want to make a disclosure at this point to erase any confusion as you read. Gerson therapy in its purest form is extremely rigid and precise. I understand that there needs to be a pure standard, one that ensures victory for the toughest cases and makes no allowances for aggressive and deadly disease to be the victor. However, reality often differs from the ideal. My story plays these shortcomings out. Therefore, I will give you a list of the ideal and my reality, so that, when you see the gaps between the two, in my entries, you will have full knowledge and understanding what the ideal really should be. Just to be clear, I was really strict with myself for the first 3 months. Also, I reference Dr. Stillings being located in Redlands, CA. He is now located in the Midwest.

Gerson Ideal	**My Reality**
No salt	Some salt, but none that I added
No oil except flax oil	Very little added oils
No non-organic food	Some non-organic food, especially out
No nuts	Very little nuts
No meat or dairy	Very little meat
No beans	Very little beans
No soaking in a tub	Attempted ginger baths
No processed food	Some organic pasta, some organic chips, some Organic hummus, etc
Green apples for drinks	Gala apples
Organic Endive	Can't find it
Organic watercress	Can't find it

No substitutes for greens	Kale, celery, collard greens, dandelions Bok Choy, spinach, mustard greens, etc.
No cocoa	Some organic dark chocolate
Hippocrates soup every day	No parsnips and no celery root and certainly Not every day
One quart of coffee for an enema	I use one cup of coffee at a strength equal to the quart.
	I also do a quick water enema before my coffee, which helps me hold my coffee

I have to say, this next section that describes my decision to learn Gerson therapy and practice it for 3 months before my return to work, takes place during the most beautiful time of the year. I end up in Redlands, CA for 10 glorious days and then am able to be at home for May, June and July. I cannot tell you how encouraging it was to be home, in a place where there was plenty of green grass and sunshine, quiet and shady country roads to walk on, birds singing and the warmth of the sun on my neck. Being in a physical paradise certainly was good for my soul. In addition, I could sleep till 8:00 every morning, had plenty of time to use my new Norwalk juicer and prepare my food throughout the day. I had no idea how luxurious that would actually be.

Rainy Day Fund

April 20, 2013

Busy, was online looking at things like hyperthermia treatment for cancer and realized my dad had this treatment to beat his melanoma 11 or 12 years ago.

AND very exciting!!! I just made my first rainy day fund expenditure on an infrared sauna. A traditional sauna uses convection heat which can get up to between 160 and 200 degrees, can't breathe and you feel like you're going to pass out. The sweat you sweat in a traditional sauna yields 97% water and 3% toxins. An infrared sauna uses infrared light to radiate your body, heating it at cooler temps and yielding sweat that is 85% water and 15%

toxins…yippee!!! Also, it is a lot more comfortable. I could go pay for these services at a spa at $50 a pop or just buy my own so I splurged…mmm, maybe a little more than what I would have spent on my trip to Greece. Had a great day out to breakfast AND the movies! And got some yard work in too. A great Day!

This verse is from my friend Reina…

Psalms 34:19

Many are the afflictions of the righteous, but the Lord delivers him out of them all.

May you feel as many taps of love as there are buds on the trees! Lynn

More Toys

April 21, 2013

Saving my life is more important than my life savings. So regardless of my short term plans, which are still up in the air, the long term plan is to be healthy and stay healthy. I purchased a few more toys. Some people buy a boat. Some people buy a four wheel RV. I just purchased a Norwalk juicer. I was going to say this is the Cadillac of juicers, but I'm betting it is the Rolls Royce of juicers. What else? Mmm…a new water distilling machine from Waterwise, because I have ALWAYS trusted enough to drink the tap water, but no more. Everything I read says, "Drink distilled water." By the time I am done with this house, I will be able to hang a sign in front, "The Ford Wellness Center" and you will be welcome to visit anytime.

Eat pure, think pure, be pure! Lots of love, Lynn

The Longevity Center

April 22, 2013

If you are curious, the place I am considering going to try to save my bladder is called The Longevity Center in Redlands CA. It is run by Dr. Donald Stillings, DC/nutritionist/homeopath. He is certified in Gerson therapy and Gerson trained. He has been practicing Gerson since about 2001 or 2 and practicing medicine for over 30 years. The setting is not a hospital, but rather like a bed and breakfast and he only has 4 guests at any one time, because this is a place where clients learn how to do Gerson therapy in a home setting so they can do it when they return to their own home.

I spent some time on the phone with his wife Janet who works there. They do have at least one case of helping someone who had bladder cancer that she remembered clearly. See, they don't treat any disease; they train people to heal their broken immune systems.

She is going to try to get more info for me about the case or other cases.

The Norwalk Juicer salesman I was directed to from the Gerson website had high praises for the Stillings...small community of practitioners.

The trick may be getting my PCP to sign the STD papers for this. I need a couple more conversations before I commit. And if I go, it will only be for 10 days.

God, grant me wisdom and please open and close doors as you see fit.

Lots of love! Lynn

Second Opinion, not Yet

April 24, 2013

Well, I went to see a new Urologist today for a second opinion. Unfortunately, my medical records were sent but were not received so he could not tell me much. Based on my understanding of my current condition, he spoke very favorably about possible options. My 1st doctor said that BCG was not still an option. This guy says it absolutely may be an option. And he said if that doesn't work, there are other avenues to try before taking my bladder out. I go back tomorrow for a scope and with medical records in hand so he can get a better idea.

I asked him if a trip to CA for 10 days is a problem. He said that would not be a problem. He can work around that. So against the judgment of family members and maybe friends too, I have made arrangements to go to The Longevity Center from May 6th to May 15th. I arrive home on the morning of the 16th. This means I have now only committed to 10 days of training which does not feel like jumping off a cliff. If bladder removal was the only choice offered, I was going to commit a longer time to Gerson therapy, taking a greater risk. (And honestly, I really think time away is a good idea!)

Hopefully tomorrow, my new doctor will give me even more encouraging news. Ironically, my CT scan is also booked for tomorrow, unfortunately AFTER my apt. with my new doctor.

This just gets curiouser and curiouser!

It bears repeating: *I can do all things through him who gives me strength.* Lots of love! Lynn

Answered Prayer

April 25, 2013

Today I had two really big prayers I put before God (about a100 times). The first prayer was for my doctor to tell me conclusively that he thinks a second shot at BCG is the way to go. This was not a given since he did not have my records yesterday and he also did a scope today. The prayer was answered as I desired. I will be doing another round of BCG. Unfortunately, he also saw more tumor in my bladder today. So I will have surgery first on May 22nd, then BCG.

The second prayer is, God please let this CT scan show no cancer outside the bladder. Still praying for that one. Will probably know the results on Tuesday when I meet with Urologist number 1.

I had a great talk with Dr. Stillings in CA about a case of advanced bladder cancer he dealt with several years ago with just Gerson therapy. The woman is doing great after 5 years. And a Naturopath friend of mine, Mark Sanders ND, said he is familiar with Gerson and thinks this is a good time for it :)

Love, love, love. The gospel in a word, is Love! Lynn

A Game of Inches

April 26, 2013

Jeep has a new commercial called, *Chip Away*. The narration is Al Pacino's speech from the movie, *Any Given Sunday* (I don't recommend the movie)

Life is a game of inches...the inches we need are everywhere around us. Every minute, every second we fight for that inch. That's all it is...every day we chip away.

For me, it's not about inches, but millimeters or smaller. Did the cancer move? Did it breech the wall? Did it breech the muscle barrier? I'm fighting to hold the line. And I'm pushing hard to gain a hair line, a fraction of a millimeter, but I'm pushing. Today, more progress in my pursuit of health, pursuit of victory...

I started the paper work for Short Term Disability. I passed my plan of attack by my PCP and she is giving her blessing to me for focused work on building my body up to fight. As soon as I get the paper work from Liberty Mutual, my PCP will submit, with May 6th, being the first day at The Longevity Center. The time period covered will be the 10 days in CA for Gerson therapy, the time for surgery and recovery and the 6 weeks for my second round of BCG. The 6 weeks will allow me the environment and time to put into practice Gerson principles in my home, and continue to augment again with yoga, aerobic exercise and infrared sauna time.

Like I said, this place is going to be like a wellness center. Just plugged in my water distiller, cool! BUT, in all my planning, I always soberly remember...God is the ONLY one who can deliver.

John 5:30

By myself I can do nothing

Inch by inch, day by day, I love you more and more, Lynn

In the Zone

April 28, 2013

As I prepare for my trip to CA, 7 days from now, I'm really trying to get in the zone. I am finally addressing the air and water quality in my home. Remember that commercial with the bottle of air and bottle of water on the porch, trying to get us to not pollute? I do. The only water I will drink or cook with at this point is distilled water (from my new cool distillery) or Poland Springs, if I can help it. I also moved a big potted plant into my bedroom to clean the air and provide more oxygen and put a high powered Sharper Image air purifier in the den where I watch TV.

And I think I am finally at the point where my perception of food has changed forever. For the first few months of my new diet, I was still always looking for the simple carbs, rice or potato or bread, chips. I still enjoy a little of that, but now I almost look for that simply for the calories so that my weight doesn't go down anymore. It's great not to have to struggle with cravings all the time. In training for detox!

...purifying my love for you!!! Lynn

Mac Daddy Juicer

April 29, 2013

It's a little like Christmas around here, maybe like the 12 days of Christmas. Two packages awaited me when I got home today. The first was a supplement called Salvestrol. There is something naturally in plants that wards off disease and pests, but this component of the plant has been manipulated out of most food we buy today by over use of herbicides and pesticides. It is believed that this component, sorry I don't know if it is a compound or enzyme, works the same way in our bodies as it does naturally in the plant. Anyway, it was recommended by my Naturopath friend Mark and I'm trying it.

The second package was also bursting with healing power! It is touted as THE best juicer in the world and I believe it. It's really big and very labor intensive. Lots of parts to clean, but it claims that with its hydraulic press I will get 55% more juice than any other juicer. Mom and I had our first glasses of carrot juice today, yum! When I emptied the waste it was almost perfectly dry! I know, it doesn't take much to excite me.

Psalm 103 by David.

Praise the Lord, my soul;
all my inmost being, praise his holy name.
Praise the Lord, my soul,
and forget not all his benefits—

*who forgives all your sins
and heals all your diseases,
who redeems your life from the pit
and crowns you with love and compassion,*

AND I feel your love and compassion too! TX, XO, Lynn

Another Answered Prayer!

April 30, 2013

Of course the bottom line is I pray for God to heal me, understood, but it is nice to hit some milestones. I was fervently praying as some of you were too, thank you, for my CT scan to come back clean of cancer outside the bladder. I love when my doc walks in with a smile on his face. Today he had a smile on his face. According to the CT scan, there is no cancer outside the bladder. Hooray!!!!

Thank you God! Off to prayer time.... Love, Lynn

Majestic Mountains

May 5, 2013

I know! It's already 9:00 there, only 6:00 here. I flew through Salt Lake City for the first time. Flying out, I looked out the window to see the most spectacular snow covered mountain peaks. I have flown a fair amount, but I think that was the most striking view I have ever seen, miles and miles of white capped mountains. Breathtaking!

Just got up from my nap. Amelia, my rock solid friend of 30 years, who is taking care of me on my trip, and I are off to dinner. We are staying in a beautiful Spanish themed hotel. The room is pure luxury. Too bad we have to leave tomorrow.

Matthew 17:20

Truly I tell you, if you have faith as small as a mustard seed, you can say to this mountain, 'Move from here to there,' and it will move. Nothing will be impossible for you.

Love you as high as the mountains, Lynn

Oops! No phone reception Day 1 at The Longevity Center

May 6, 2013

Well, I guess it is a really good thing that I brought my laptop because I have absolutely no phone reception here at all. Please don't think I am neglecting you or ignoring you. I did get just a couple texts, but the phone dies if I get a call and I did have texts that I tried to send, fail. Maybe I am meant to have more quiet time than I was planning on.... :)

Lots of love, Lynn

In school, Day 2 at The Longevity Center

May 7, 2013

My mother always teases me, calling me the eternal student, not in a complimentary way. She says I was in college for 10 years. I think it was really 8 years if you don't count time taken off. Of late, I LOVE learning the science behind the workings of our bodies and how food and other things interact with our bodies. Here I get to sit at the feet of Dr. Stillings as he passionately explains how things really work. I said I could listen to him all day and he said, "that's because this rings true." Much like reading the Bible is for me. The more you read, the more it rings true and somehow, finding truth is so exciting.

Today we learned about the supplements we need to take while on the Gerson therapy, things we need and do not get enough of, for instance, Pancreatin. Yeah, I've never heard of it before either. It is an enzyme that our bodies make in the pancreas, but as we get older our body loses its ability to make as much as we can use. This helps. Yesterday and today are the first days I've ever learned anything about the importance of enzymes. Something new every day!!

This is the scripture my new friend Bronwyn shared with me today:

Hebrews 4:15

For we have not an high priest [Jesus] which cannot be touched with the feeling of our infirmities; but was in all points tempted like as we are, yet without sin. Let us therefore come boldly unto the throne of grace, that we may obtain mercy, and find grace to help in time of need. (This might be the King James Version)

Loving you, in any version! Lynn

Day 3 at The Longevity Center

May 8, 2013

Busy, busy, busy! Today we learned more about supplements we need to take and about "healing reactions." Healing reactions is a nice way of saying, you are going to get sick before you get well. Just like when someone goes to drug rehab and detox and has withdrawal and detox episodes, I will too! These episodes should come in the form of nausea or flu like symptoms. The doc said they can last from 6 hours to 3 days. They are worse in the first 3 months than later, but are necessary for healing.

Amelia and her cousin Allie came for a visit today. It does my soul good. She will be back on Saturday with Janice, another old friend from Massasoit Community College. Fantastic!! The sun was out and hot today while we were driving around Redlands, but once we stepped outside to sit in the garden the clouds returned and it was chilly again. The sun has to come out eventually.

2 Samuel 22:2

The Lord is my rock, my fortress and my deliverer.

Still love you even if I'm three hours late (away), Lynn

Day 4 at The Longevity Center

May 9, 2013

Today during a short break, Bronwyn, Juanita and I went for a stroll in the neighborhood. It is amazing to me that everyone has glorious flowers in their yard. Almost every yard has roses. Then there are large spires of trees. I have no idea what they are called, but they are 30 feet tall, plus Palm trees, Willow, Cedar all kinds of conifers and just a crazy variety of all sorts of flowers that I have never seen before. It is lovely here, probably 70 degrees today. Today our morning lesson was on PH. Every day we learn about something different and Dr. Stillings says each day that whatever we are looking at, "There is a whole discipline just devoted to this."

Five more minutes till my next drink. I just finished my lunch. Then I have 2 hours. Definitely will take a nap today. Was up late last night playing with clay packs.

To God be the glory! Love you! Lynn

The Proof is in the Pudding, Day 5 at The Longevity Center

May 10, 2013

Last night we got to watch a video of Charlotte Gerson giving a lecture at a conference. At the time, she was just turning 70. She is now in her 90s or there about. Of course when she speaks, everything she says about Gerson therapy makes perfect sense. She is not an MD, but is thoroughly familiar with all the ins and outs of her father's, (Max Gerson) work. She was fielding questions like a trained physician, but I think she is able to do that because the therapy and the principles of the therapy are so simple in nature.

Anyway, she is certainly convincing, but even more convincing is the state of her physical health. She said she dropped her health insurance when she was 46 years old or 46 years ago, not only because she never used it, but didn't want any procedures her insurance was going to offer. She said she has never even had a mammogram. Plus she had person after person after person, fascinating cases, stand up and share their stories. Simply, the proof is in the pudding.

Matthew 7:17-18

Likewise, every good tree bears good fruit, but a bad tree bears bad fruit. A good tree cannot bear bad fruit, and a bad tree cannot bear good fruit.

She is a good tree, the tree I want to be! Lots of love, Lynn

Reunion Today, Day 6 at The Longevity Center

May 11, 2013

Today Amelia came to visit with our old friend Janice. We were all in a Bible study group at Massassoit Community College in 1983. WOWZA! These women are THE salt of the earth! Never changing, solid in their love!

K, love you! Lynn

Day 7 at The Longevity Center

May 12, 2013

Yesterday, I made an attempt to up my game by implementing the full Gerson Protocol. That's 13 drinks, 5 coffee enemas, plus supplements. It was a very busy day, cooking demonstration, plus lecture, plus instructional video, plus company!!! I did 13 drinks, plus 4 enemas. I guess it is important to note, that my company here tells me that what we are doing is not a colonic. When doing an enema, I only insert my hose in an inch or so. During a colonic, a tube, called a speculum, is inserted deeper into the colon. After warm water is flushed in, the water is flushed back out creating suction. This goes back and forth for about an hour. What I do is not painful or difficult and lasts only 15 minutes. A quick water enema before the coffee helps clean me out and better hold my coffee.

Today, I saw on my schedule, the addition of 2 tablespoons of castor oil.... yuck!! I was pleasantly surprised to find that it does not really have any taste at all, certainly not like the dreaded Cod Liver oil. However, it still does not go down easily. And of course, the not going down easily was the easy part. I don't think the castor oil is critical to the success of the therapy. If not, I think I'll skip this going forward.

If you are thinking of watching one of the Gerson documentaries, I liked, *The Gerson Miracle* best.

I'm loving the miracle of your love for me! Lots of love, Lynn

Day 8 at The Longevity Center

May 13, 2013

Upping my game is not as easy as I thought it would be. The castor oil treatment made me feel sick yesterday, as expected, but today, every time I stood up, I felt like I was going to black out and my tummy still hurt today. The tummy trouble may be left over from the castor oil. The Dr. says the castor oil works so well to clean out your system because the body sees it as foreign, not something it wants to keep in the body so it tries to eliminate it as quickly as possible. The benefit is that it pulls lots of toxins out with it. I asked the Dr. about being light headed and he said we have turned my body into a 3 shift factory so it is working really hard round the clock to be nourished and detox. Even though I am getting more nourished and less toxic, there are big goings on inside and it takes a toll.

I am already anticipating my last day and already miss being here. I have felt like this is home even from the first day. Part of my desire not to leave is the trek around the world I have to make to get home. It will be 11 hours of flight time alone and another 3.5 hours in airports. Plus with all the work being done by the Dr.'s wife Jan, it is really like being on vacation. At home, I will be in the kitchen ALOT.

Well, more to do, more to do....save up your hugs for me, xo, Lynn

Day 9 at The Longevity Center

May 14, 2013

Today we continued our important discussion on enzymes. There are 23 digestive enzymes and over 10,000 metabolic enzymes!! See, now you are as smart as a 5th grader! I am doing much better today. No racing to the girls' room, no light headedness :)

We took a walk to the top of the street and could see the beautiful San Bernadino mountain range all around us and took plenty of pictures. Nap time!

1 Corinthians 10:31

So whether you eat or drink or whatever you do, do it all for the glory of God.

Looking forward to breaking bread with you!!! Love, Lynn

Day 10 at The Longevity Center

May 15, 2013

Alrighty! Today is my last day with Dr. Stillings and his superwoman wife Jan. They make a terrific team. They have made our stay the very best it could be. I can't imagine what else they could have done or been to make our stay better. They are the perfect host and hostess. They are from the Midwest originally and will be moving their operation back there in August so they can be more accessible to the nation. Their homespun goodness is through and through.

It has also been a tremendous blessing to be here with good souls from the south, Juanita and her daughter Bronwyn, from Mississippi and Louisiana respectively. They have been my constant companions here 12 and 13 hours a day. We walk together, eat and drink together, pray together, learn together, laugh and encourage one another. "Bless their hearts."... I fear I will have trouble getting rid of my new accent and don't be surprised if I bless your heart.

Amelia will make one more, long trek from Palos Verdes to gather me up and deliver me to the airport. I fly overnight and arrive in Providence at about 9:30 tomorrow morning. My friend Constance will gather me up from the airport and deliver me to my reliable Corolla for the journey home.

There will be a lot to do to set up my kitchen and stock my kitchen when I get home, but now I have the tools and confidence to believe I can do this one way or another for the two years prescribed for all cancer patients. That's right, TWO YEARS!

On my way to see you...whom I love, Lynn

Home Sweet Home

May 16, 2013

Wow! I flew all night, got home and slept for a few hours. Such a headache I have! Of course, my routine is all thrown off. I made it through the first gauntlet, 15 hours of travel and the only thing I put in my mouth from the airport was Smart Water and gum. I had raw veggies and boiled potato in my back pack. I had tomato juice on the plane. I ate some peanut butter when I got home, which is not on my diet.

People always ask me what I eat. My choices just got really narrow. I am now limited to organic veggies and fruit, a little flax seed or coconut oil and rye, seedless bread, or sprouted bread, but there is also an additional list of things I cannot have. That means I am now cutting out all beans, nuts and seeds, nut milks and nut butters as well as all berries, mushrooms and cucumbers and pineapple.

I only lost 2 lbs in the last 10 days. I weigh 118. Okay, my number one goal every day will be to make sure I have clean (organic) food and clean (distilled) water. That means I have to run to the grocery store to eat supper!! Love you!!!
Lynn

My Mantra

May 17, 2013

Okay, I have discovered that my mantra is, "There has got to be a better way!" That's why I am doing Gerson therapy to begin with. I looked at was being offered and decided that there had to be a better way to heal. What I was offered was not even healing. Today I went for a visit with Urologist # 2 who will be performing my surgery on the 22nd. The visit was about 10 minutes long. Kind of went like this, "Do you have any questions?" To which I replied, "No." It took almost an hour and a half to get there and, no lie, 3 hours exactly to get home. There has GOT to be a better way!

I am going to insist that they don't schedule an appointment unless absolutely needed. That seems reasonable. What would be more reasonable would be for insurance to pay for a phone consult. How do sick people do it??? Warning: Don't ever get sick!!!

...baby steps. Today I went food shopping for the week, but did not actually get everything on the list, $198.00 at Whole Foods. I pulled out my list and was very overwhelmed. I felt like I was shopping for a small restaurant. Yes, I realize I will have to shop around. I was able to get 10% off a 50 lb. bag of organic carrots. I managed to get 4 juiced drinks in today and no detox due to equipment breakage. I will however take a ginger bath. That should or maybe induce either a fever or at least profuse sweating...until my sauna is put together.

Can't remember how the song goes, but "My God is so big, so mighty and strong! There's nothing my God cannot do!!"

Loving you as much today as yesterday, but maybe even more tomorrow!! Lynn

Training for the Olympics

May 18, 2013

It is starting to sink in...what this Gerson therapy really means for my life. I told my Mom today and am telling you now, my commitment to Gerson therapy will be like training for the Olympics for the next two years. Not that I have ever trained for the Olympics, but that is the best my brain could come up with. If a person training for the Olympics has to go to school or go to work that means, probably up at 4:00 or 5:00, one or two hours of training before work, then a few hours of training after work and then to bed early. Everything of no value, (meaning anything that doesn't get me closer to Gold) will be stripped out of my schedule. Special diet, strict bed time, money is tight...all resources are accounted for and all focus is on the GOLD.

I am not choosing two years randomly. Two years is the Gerson protocol for any cancer patient. Yup, I'm way in deep now. But this is what I believe will not only heal my cancer but all things disease like. My CT scan from November shows a cyst in my liver, a cyst in my left kidney, an enlarged uterus, even a little atherosclerosis (plaque in my veins). Now that the docs have their hands on me they want me to go to the gynecologist, want me to make an apt with the dermatologist, want me to make an apt with the hematologist, take an MRI of my kidney. I have the CT scan from November and the CT scan from April. Already, my 1st Urologist told my mom that the cyst in my kidney was smaller than 5 months ago. That change is just from being on the Fuhrman diet for 5 months. The Gerson diet will accelerate good changes so I can make my escape from allopathic medicine.

Allopathic medicine is an expression commonly used by homeopaths and proponents of other forms of alternative medicine to refer to mainstream medical use of pharmacologically active agents or physical interventions to treat or suppress symptoms or pathophysiologic processes of diseases or conditions. -Wikipedia

I love the idea of medical freedom! Also, the freedom to love you! Lynn

Stumbling out of the blocks

May 19, 2013

Today was day 14 of 730. That's how I see it. It was also the first day I ventured outside of my house still with the goal of doing all 10 of my juices. I packed two carrot juices in a to-go cup and went to church which was an outdoor service at Franklin Park. I got out of friend Brian's snazzy red Wrangler and discovered that my pant leg was wet. I checked my to-go cup and found it to be empty! Empty in my shoulder bag :(There I was in the middle of the park, on my knees, dumping the carrot soaked contents of my bag into the grass. It was not the mess that was discouraging, but the fact that I just lost all the precious liquid gold. Heartbreaking, I tell you. But, we had a great service and I got home and just decided that even though I was way behind, I would just make it up. There is a will and there is a way!

Also, Dr. Dave, the bestest pediatrician in the world was concerned about where my calcium is coming from and if I am getting enough. There is more calcium in a cup of Bok Choy then a cup of milk and 54% of the calcium in the Bok Choy will be absorbed whereas only 32% of the calcium in the milk will be absorbed. Now I am not eating 3 or 4 cups of Bok Choy each day, but I am eating Bok Choy each day as well as other high calcium veggies, like broccoli, chard, and cabbage. Also, I drink orange juice which is also high in calcium. Plus, I am getting over 400 mg of calcium just from carrot juice and drinking 3 green juices as well. I'm pretty sure my calcium needs are being met. Thanks for the concern Dr. Dave!

To do: buy a thermos!

Lots of love, Lynn

The Thrill of Victory

May 21, 2013

I always say that victory comes in small pieces. Today I made the long trek into Beth Israel to see a couple nice docs. Much ado about nothing, but I got to use my new thermos!! I consumed 3 juiced drinks in transit and was able to complete my required 10 drinks for the day. Next time I will need to remember to bring all the accompanying supplements. I don't just take supplements once in the morning. I take some with every drink. It's a lot.

Be safe out there kids! Love, Lynn

Surgery Today

May 22, 2013

Just got home from the hospital. Had my 4th transurethral resection of the bladder tumor (TURBT), I think that's what it's called, cleaning the cancer cells out of my bladder. The good news, the doc said there was very little to remove.

Hopefully, I heal for 3 to 4 weeks then we try a second round of BCG. Six weeks of that and then more healing, then biopsy.

My hope is that Joel Fuhrman's nutrient dense diet has held the line, meaning that is has kept the cancer from passing into the muscle AND that Gerson therapy will actually help turn the tide and help my body to start defeating the cancer in the bladder.

With the combination of the Gerson and BCG I think I have good odds, all under the umbrella of God. In the meantime, more fun with catheters!

I love loving you! Lynn

An Apple a Day?

May 24, 2013

How about 7 apples a day? That's how many I go through each day on Gerson therapy. I drink 3 green drinks. There is an apple in each one. Then I mix apple juice with 4 of my carrot drinks, 7 a day. But carrots are what I consume the most of, about 6 or 7 lbs of carrots a day, well, the juice of 6 or 7 lbs. Now you are getting the idea of what kind of nutrient load it may take to make up for the nutrient deficiency in my body.

Is all of this really needed? Not many people have claimed to be able to cure cancer. Dr. Max Gerson did make that claim and he did it with massive amounts of nutrition and an equal amount of detox. Since this is not an easy program, I'm sure he would not have prescribed more than what he understood it would take to do the job.

Even Joel Fuhrman says in one of his videos that as a species we should be getting 10 times the amount of nutrients that we, Americans typically get, so Max Gerson's ideas seem to make sense.

Did I mention? The juice bar is open. If you stop by I'll make a fresh glass for you. I think fresh squeezed apple juice is really yummy! If you choose to bring your own apples, I understand that Delicious are not good for juicing, FYI, or you can have a green or carrot juice!

I raise my glass to you! Lots of love, Lynn

Christmas in a Box

May 25, 2013

I've been home more than a week now and my Christmas in a box has been waiting for me in the garage since my return. Can you imagine getting to Christmas morning and finding a box in your living room stamped, "Open in 9 days?" That's what it has felt like waiting for my sauna to be assembled. My fabulous brothers, Mark and Steven, are slated to put it together tomorrow at 9:00. It will not be an easy job. We, (they), have to rearrange gym equipment in the basement to make room. Mom's Power Plate has to be moved and the tread mill has to be moved. Then the sauna will be taken down through the bulkhead in 3 pieces. Assembled it will weigh over 400 lbs. I can't wait. Could definitely use it tonight. It is only 42 degrees outside.

Just a reminder: EVERY thing I do is focused on eliminating cancer from my body. The fewer toxins in my body, the better my body will fight the cancer. Usually, I would leave carrots for Santa's reindeer, but from now on, I'm leaving carrot juice for Santa!

Nothing says Christmas like being with you! Love, Lynn

Laborers of Love

May 26, 2013

Mark and Steven put together my sauna today. I will try it out tonight. It took a couple hours. I suggested that it would be more fun than building a model car, but I don't think they were biting. Later in the afternoon, friend June came by with 3 or 4 trays of Impatience. We typically fill our flower boxes on the north side of the house with them. She cheerfully planted, careful to arrange with a color pattern, then filled the box on the cabana and then planted around the huge red Maple tree in the front yard. My friend Beth had come by a few weeks ago and filled one flower box with mini Snap Dragons and some other beautiful filler, Silver Fox or something. She also filled all our hanging plants in the back with Pansies. Everything is blooming nicely, adding luscious color to our otherwise very green landscape.

Hey, there are definitely perks and upsides to having a serious illness. Don't let anyone tell you otherwise. Theses laborers of love take the edge off of life's demands, but more than that confirm their love for me in seriously concrete ways. But no one can compete with Mom, who endures the churning and grinding of my juicer from 8:00 in the morning until 2:00 in the afternoon. Then she cleans up after me, all day long, even indignant if I suggest otherwise. I experience the love God has for me through every kind gesture, every kind text and every kind act. As Jewel says, "We are his hands, we are his eyes."

Hoping at this twilight hour that your day was a great one, just like mine!!! Lots of love to you!! Lynn

Paring Down

May 27, 2013

I am realizing the true cost of Gerson! I can only do one short jaunt from home each day and still accomplish my goal. Yesterday I had to choose between a guest at my house or the neighbor's cookout. Today I had to choose between a shopping trip with my Mom or a friend's engagement party. Gerson may take a huge toll on me in terms of my social life. I already knew that, but now I am living it. The very hardest thing is I literally cannot go out to eat, ANY WHERE! If you know of any organic restaurants on the south shore, please be sure to let me know, or any restaurants that may have organic offerings on the menu.

This will be an interesting summer!!! ...still, going for the gold medal in health!!

Of course my goal for gold, is to share all my training secrets with you!! Lots of love, Lynn

Biopsy Results/Status

May 28, 2013

The Dr. called with biopsy results from my surgery on May 22nd. He said he removed very little which to me indicates that there probably was very little to no growth since Urologist #1 was in there on April 9th. YAY! The problem is the cancer there is still high grade, just not a lot of it. So we wait 3 weeks and start BCG. In some cases, when the first round of BCG doesn't work, interferon is added with the BCG, but my urologist says it is not really effective, so we are just going with the BCG again...BCG and my secret weapon, Gerson therapy.

Status: Dr. Stillings says that my body temp should be at 97 degrees to fight cancer. I have not been able to get my basil temp (lowest temp of the day) to 97. I have been juicing religiously, detoxing too! I have not eaten or drunk anything I shouldn't. However, surgery may have hindered my goal. Also, I have not been exercising, so I added a 30 minute walk to my day, starting today. That should help. I also have not been able to use my sauna consistently. I used it once. I will shoot for 2 or 3 times a week through the end of my BCG treatments. This will accelerate detox and speed the strengthening of my immune system. Also, cancer does not like heat. Hyperthermia is a known killer of cancer cells.

Okay, settling into the trenches for the big battle! Love being in the trenches with you! Thanks for your support! Love, Lynn

Purging the Aluminum

May 29, 2013

I just happen to live in the house where my father grew up. It was built in 1931 by my grandfather and is beautifully built, rock solid. In addition to having its original everything, I think some of the items in the draws and cabinets are also original. For instance, our kitchen is filled with aluminum gadgets with wooden handles, some red and some green. They look like they are from 1931. The Gerson book says to get rid of all aluminum cookware because the aluminum will leach into your food. So we have begun the purge. Let's see, to start, a hand held mill that Mom used to make pasta fagoli with. She would press the kidney beans through to get just the meat of the beans. We also used this to make applesauce. We found a hand held "ricer". I think we used this to make mashed potatoes. Oh yeah, and the masher we used on potato and butternut squash; also all the grates for grating and a small hand held grater. I'm sure we will find more. We have begun replacing with stainless steel. We will all be safer for it! Dr. Stillings told me about a trick. Take a magnet with you when you shop for your stainless steel. A magnet will not stick to stainless steel. Cool huh!

Sat in the sauna for the second time last night. It worked better this time. Slept like a baby :)

Here is a quote sent to me by Bridget, a faith filled woman.

Isaiah 40:28-31

The Lord is the everlasting God,
    the Creator of the ends of the earth.
He will not grow tired or weary,
    and his understanding no one can fathom.
He gives strength to the weary
    and increases the power of the weak.
Even youths grow tired and weary,
    and young men stumble and fall;
but those who hope in the Lord
    will renew their strength.

They will soar on wings like eagles;
   they will run and not grow weary,
   they will walk and not be faint.

Hoping you put your hope in the Lord and soar like eagles, love, Lynn

Getting my Priorities Straight

May 31, 2013

The good Dr. Stillings said it would take a couple weeks to get into the Gerson routine. I think I'm almost there. I have to be vigilant about guarding my schedule. I can lose valuable juicing time REALLY easily and then it can be hard to catch up. And I have to have conviction as hard as a rock. Here are my new priorities:

1. My relationship with God, through reading, prayer, church, fellowship

2. Now, 12 fresh raw juices a day, including 4 green drinks and 8 carrot/apple drinks.

3. Now, 4 coffee enemas a day

4. Only organic veggies and fruit for meals

5. All my Gerson recommended supplements. (A lot!)

6. A 30 minute walk each day

7. 30 minutes in the sauna every other day, for now

8. Expressing my unending gratitude for all my blessings, most of whom are PEOPLE!

9. Continuing to connect with you!

I think I will stay in Psalms for a while. When you need to address the needs of self, Psalms is a good place to set a while.

Psalm 23:1-6

The Lord is my shepherd, I lack nothing.
  He makes me lie down in green pastures,
he leads me beside quiet waters,
  he refreshes my soul.
He guides me along the right paths
  for his name's sake.
Even though I walk
  through the darkest valley,
I will fear no evil,
  for you are with me;
your rod and your staff,
  they comfort me.
You prepare a table before me
  in the presence of my enemies.
my cup overflows.
You anoint my head with oil;
Surely your goodness and love will follow me
  all the days of my life,
    and I will dwell in the house of the Lord
  forever.

Hope to dwell there with you!!! Lots of love, Lynn

Hippocrates Soup for You

June 1, 2013

The question I get lately is, "Are you only juicing and not eating anything?" The answer is I am juicing, but I am also eating 3 meals a day. I am allowed organic oatmeal in the morning. I find that raisins make it plenty sweet enough, yum! Then at lunch and dinner it is recommended that I eat salad, soup and a couple cooked, hot veggies, like potato or squash to cushion all the raw food my belly is dealing with. The soup most served at the Gerson facility is called, Hippocrates Soup. This is it:

1 medium celery knob or 3 or 4 stalks of celery
2 small leeks
2 medium onions
A little parsley
1 medium parsnip
Garlic as desired
1 or 2 tomatoes
1 or 2 potatoes

Do not peel. Wash, cut coarsely, cover in a saucepan with distilled water, simmer 2 hours, (or just cook till tender), put through food mill, done.

Note: putting it through a food mill is too much work for me and I don't care for so much liquid so I just cover halfway, cook till tender, then mash it with a masher. It's thick and yummy! I added some cauliflower today. I like it :) What is so special about this soup? Leeks, onion and garlic are really high on the list of cancer fighting foods, cauliflower too!!

As many of you know, it is said that Hippocrates said, "Let food be thy medicine."

Food and thoughts of you are my medicine! Love, Lynn

Let Me Implore You

June 2, 2013

One friend said this week. "I've made some changes, but I'm not where you are." Another said, "Are you trying to convert this guy to your diet?" My answer to both comments was that I don't wish this diet on anyone.

Gerson therapy is just that, therapy, though very long term therapy. I was just adapting to Joel Fuhrman's "Nutritarian Diet" and I jumped to this. As I noted before, this is isolating. I feel like I'm a girl in a bubble.

I once said that getting bladder cancer is kind of like getting a new puppy. There are new out of pocket expenses, some juggling with my schedule, lots more demands on my time and resources. Well, if getting bladder cancer is like getting a new puppy, then doing Gerson therapy is like getting a new baby, with the exception that I actually get to sleep at night. This is VERY expensive, hours and hours of my day are consumed, I can barely get out to do anything without lots of planning and I don't expect much breathing room in the next two years.

So If you haven't heard me yet, let me implore you, take care of your health now! Respect your freedom. I know, I know!! It's hard, but when you lose your health, you lose all freedom. You put yourself in danger of financial hardship, or losing your job or career! Just do this; KEEP learning, be vested in your health and make small changes that will add up quickly. Do NOT count on the gym to keep you healthy. Exercise is important, but it alone will NOT keep you healthy. If Lance Armstrong can get cancer, anyone can.

Need a suggestion? Significantly reduce dairy and meat products. Chances are you are getting way too much animal protein. Hey, it's summer time, put some veggies on the grill! Have another slice of watermelon.

From my bubble to you, lots of love!!! Lynn

Going REALLY Green

June 6, 2013

Four of my twelve drinks each day are green drinks prescribed by my Gerson therapy. The recipe calls for:

Romaine lettuce (3 large leaves)
Swiss Chard (1 big leaf)
Beet greens
Watercress
Red cabbage
A quarter of a green pepper
Endive
Escarole
An apple
Red leaf lettuce

We currently have 3 fridges going. All my greens are kept in the fridge in the garage. I take a basket, the size of a shoe box (child's shoes) and trek out to the fridge. I fill my basket and then it's to the kitchen to juice. It is literally enough food for a good sized salad! A month ago, I couldn't even tell you what endive looked like, or watercress, or chard! I still can't tell you what escarole looks like.

I also need lots of other greens for fresh salad that I eat for lunch and dinner. Last summer I had the honor of working for Pete and Lynn Reading at Billingsgate Farm in Plympton on Rte 106. I visited there today and hit the jackpot. Whole Foods will sell me a small bunch of red leaf lettuce for $2.49. Today I bought red leaf from Lynn for $2.50 and the head of lettuce was equal to 3 or 4 heads at Whole Foods! I guess I'll be visiting Billingsgate a lot this summer. If you are in the area, check them out. They are open 7 days a week, 10:00 to 6:30, maybe 9:00 to 6:00 on Saturday and Sunday. Please support your local farmer wherever you are. Otherwise, we won't have any to support!

Psalm 25:4-5

Show me your ways, Lord,
 teach me your paths.
Guide me in your truth and teach me,
 for you are God my Savior,
 and my hope is in you all day long.

God, please show US, teach US, guide US! Lots of love, Lynn

Selective Reading

June 8, 2013

When I was at The Longevity Center in CA, my housemate, Bronwyn and I talked about how awesome it would be to open similar teaching centers in our own states of Louisiana and Massachusetts. In thinking about that kind of work I wondered if that famous scripture I've read about 500 times, about the sheep and the goats, said anything about serving sick people. I, sincerely, had wiped my mind clean of any knowledge about that.

Matthew 25:34-36

Then the King will say to those on his right, 'Come, you who are blessed by my Father; take your inheritance, the kingdom prepared for you since the creation of the world. For I was hungry and you gave me something to eat, I was thirsty and you gave me something to drink, I was a stranger and you invited me in, I needed clothes and you clothed me, I was sick and you looked after me, I was in prison and you came to visit me.'

As an advocate for the poor and needy I have always dismissed, "I was sick and you looked after me," I guess because I wanted to excuse myself...I want it to say, "and you healed me," so that I can say that verse applies to someone else, like a doctor. But, it just says, "you looked after me," so I guess it applies to me...hmmmm, now how am I going to get around, "I was in prison and you came to visit me?"

Ok, ok! If you get sick or picked up by the police, feel free to call! In fact, PLEASE call so I can check these boxes off, wink, wink! Love you, no matter what condition you are in, Lynn

Idle Capacity

June 11, 2013

I keep thinking about this wind turbine on rte. 53 in Hanover. Every time I pass it, there it sits, perfectly still. I was so excited to see it go up, months and months ago, but there it sits, perfectly still. It is disheartening to me, to see all that incredible capacity, completely idle. So much of life can be like that wind turbine...a man or woman trying to provide for the needs of the family, but unemployed, unable to find a good job; a child who cannot read or write well; a teen disengaged or caught up in drugs; an abandoned building causing more problems than good.

What do I care? It's not my money invested in that wind turbine. Do we not all prosper when the blades are turning, when the time card is punched, when a child reads to a sibling or writes a letter to the president? Do we not all prosper when the teen is on the ball field inspiring his teammates or a building is converted into a small place of business? I am always reminded how connected we are, how very connected we are. And too, I am forced to ask, how much idle capacity or potential remains in me?

Plenty of capacity for loving you! Lynn

Go in the Strength you Have

June 12, 2013

Alright I admit it! There are clothes all over my bed, some clean, some not, not sure how they got mixed. My dresser top is a mess, my desk is even a bigger mess. I haven't looked at my finances in 2 weeks. My bathroom is not presentable in the least. The downstairs bathroom, that guests actually used, was certainly not presentable at the time they used it. There is business I need to attend to, volunteer business, but business all the same. I really should clean up my email account. The blueberry bushes are still only half covered, although I have the netting in the breezeway. I hide my nails in church because they look like I've been working in the garden. Really, they are only discolored from juicing. I guess I should wear gloves. Sometimes, I leave the house to do errands and my shirt is covered with carrot juice spray. And every day before 2:00 pm the white kitchen cabinets and floor look like Jackson Pollack art work, green and orange.

However!!!! I am doing exactly what I need to be doing and when I fall short even of what I need to be doing, I am reminded of a scripture that gives me hope. In the book of Judges, chapter 6, the Lord tells Gideon to rise up and save Israel from the Midianites. Gideon protests, saying in effect, I am the least of my clan, how can I? The Lord tells him simply, "Go in the strength you have. I will be with you." This is all we can do on any given day, just go in the strength that we have and trust that God will make up the difference, as we follow him.

God and you give me the strength I have. Lots of love and gratitude, Lynn

Carcinogens Hiding

June 14, 2013

Well, my brother Steve was working in the garage today with some mighty strong commercial glue as he was constructing counter tops. As I stepped into the breezeway, I thought the fumes were going to knock me over. I opened the door to the garage and commented, "Steve, I can feel the brain damage already beginning." He replied, "Yes, drain bamage, drain bamage." You see my point. Toxins are everywhere! Be aware! Be alert to the thieves stalking you. They want to steal your health and like the cancer cells within, they have no compassion and no empathy.

Lots of pure, clean, healthy love to you! Lynn

Glorious! Glorious!

June 15, 2013

Wow! I can't believe I slept 11 hours last night with just one little short interruption. I could have lingered longer. That means I was way behind this morning. I missed time with Drew and the ladies in Marshvegas this morning and had to skip valued time with Linda and Beti tonight. Gerson definitely takes a toll on relationships.

I finally took my 10:30 walk a little after 3:00. My house is just one house from Gorham Ave, here in Pembroke. Gorham Ave is a really quiet street lined with small, neat ranches and capes. I passed the chickens and their strutting cock a doodle doo and passed as well, precious little gardens diligently attended to. This is a shady street with yards lush with Hostas and Myrtle. At the end, I turned onto Fairview which runs alongside Great Sandy Bottom Pond, hence, the fair view. I breathed in the ocean of oxygen thrown from the 30 and 40 foot Pines and Oaks. Occasionally, I saw a well-placed Japanese Red Maple. I saw a small, but spectacular white Dogwood in full bloom. Traffic is always rare and the most noise I heard was from the birds. I never tire of the crisp blue sky against the green tree tops. It was just above 70 degrees and the sun warmed my back as I walked. Afterward, I drove to the farm, just 10 minutes away. Folks were out picking strawberries. The corn in the field is about half way there. All the promise of a glorious summer to come!

Psalm 145:5

They speak of the glorious splendor of your majesty—and I will meditate on your wonderful works.

Meditating on his glorious splendor and his wonderful work in YOU! Lots of love, Lynn

A Dark Past, a Dark Cast

June 17, 2013

I took a ride to Randolph today and saw some shady characters from my past while I was out and about. There he stood, bold and brazen, with his fur trimmed coat and his gold bling, Burger King himself. We shared more than a few chicken sandwiches together. We used to meet on Adams St. in Quincy. I would meet him after work. Then I ran into that Taco Bell Chihuahua, with his big brown eyes. He whispered to me as I passed by, "You know you want a chalupa, Baby." Come on, what is more seductive than the sound of, "Chalupa... chalupaaaa?" Nothing! I thought I was out of harm's way when I ran into Wendy, just standing there with her double bacon cheese burger, juices dripping, just oozing and dripping. No sooner did I escape her, I ran into the colonel, Harland to me, all dressed in his spit and shine white suit, a devil in a white suit. I gave into his original recipe more than once. Luckily I wasn't often in his neighborhood.

But then, I never make it home without seeing him, the worst influence on me ever appeared. He's always so smug, with that fiendish grin on his face. That's right, Ronald McDonald. We were together for decades. I started seeing him when I was just a teen. We were together all the time in college. By my early 30s he had me hooked on some pretty hard stuff. I was chain diet Coking, high on fries and more often than not, strung out on Big Macs. As I neared 40, I had cleaned up some, had weaned myself off the hard stuff, but was still meeting him for breakfast on the way to church and often stopping for Happy Meals when I had the chance. Well, I just drove right by, like I do every day, but let me tell you, he broke my heart and I think it will never be mended. I'll always have a place in my soul that cannot be filled with anything else, but special sauce on a sesame seed bun.

Seeing a new guy now, Max Gerson. Unfortunately, celery knob just doesn't do it for me.

Satiated only by the company of characters like you. Love, Lynn

Wall Building

June 20, 2013

I drove to the farm today because I was in great need of lettuce. Billingsgate Farm has been getting all my lettuce business lately. Last year there were stone workers who had started building a wall along the roadside of the corn field. This wall is no joke. I would say it is maybe 3 feet wide and maybe 3 feet tall. When completed, it will be longer than a football field. I saw two guys there working today. They stood at the gap between finished wall and an 80 foot long pile of rocks. There is no mortar used. Each stone is meticulously placed and all 3 edges of the wall are completely flat. I can't even imagine the patience and focus it would take to build that wall.

Everything in our society is so fast and such a problem if it is not. I think focus and patience are lost qualities today. I like to think I have a fair amount of both, but know that I really don't. I started learning Greek and feared that even though I paid out of pocket for Rosetta Stone, I would lose my patience and give up, which is what I did. And who wants to focus on any one thing when there are sooooo many things we can do!!!!! This is a real struggle for me every day. There are so many things I want to do, but I need to focus on this defensive wall I am building to improve and protect my health. Every day I lay a few more stones and need to, until I have an impenetrable fortress completed.

So, I ask you, what have you been building lately? Is it something that will last for the ages? Or maybe you dream of beginning a wall but just haven't started.

Maybe it is too overwhelming. The funny thing is, no matter how big or small, all stone walls are built the same way, one stone at a time.

I love this story in Nehemiah 4 about the Israelites rebuilding the walls of their city, years after they had been demolished by the Babylonians. At the time of the rebuilding they also faced opposition....

6 So we rebuilt the wall till all of it reached half its height, for the people worked with all their heart...

10 Meanwhile, the people in Judah said, "The strength of the laborers is giving out, and there is so much rubble that we cannot rebuild the wall."

11 Also our enemies said, "Before they know it or see us, we will be right there among them and will kill them and put an end to the work..."

13 Therefore I stationed some of the people behind the lowest points of the wall at the exposed places, posting them by families, with their swords, spears and bows. 14 After I looked things over, I stood up and said to the nobles, the officials and the rest of the people, "Don't be afraid of them. Remember the Lord, who is great and awesome, and fight for your families, your sons and your daughters, your wives and your homes..."

16 From that day on, half of my men did the work, while the other half were equipped with spears, shields, bows and armor. The officers posted themselves behind all the people of Judah 17 who were building the wall. Those who carried materials did their work with one hand and held a weapon in the other, 18 and each of the builders wore his sword at his side as he worked...

21 So we continued the work with half the men holding spears, from the first light of dawn till the stars came out. 22 At that time I also said to the people, "Have every man and his helper stay inside Jerusalem at night, so they can serve us as guards by night and as workers by day." 23 Neither I nor my brothers nor my men nor the guards with me took off our clothes; each had his weapon, even when he went for water."

The wall was finished in spite of great opposition outside the camp and great doubt even among the builders.

Building what counts with you! Love, Lynn

Unmatched Kindness

June 22, 2013

While I was out with a friend yesterday, I had a delivery at my home. Coworker Brandi had stopped by with a card signed by many friends at work. That was a very kind gesture all on its own, but in addition, there was a very generous gift certificate to my favorite farm, Billingsgate in Plympton, that I have been telling you about. Today I made my trek to the farm and pulled out the gift certificate. Proprietor Lynn Reading said, "Oh, you are the one!" She said in all their time selling produce, no one has ever asked to buy a gift certificate. So my coworkers have set precedence, a new and wonderful idea! Instead of getting a loved one an iTunes card, or Lowes card or a gift card to a local restaurant, how about something even better? Fresh, local, organic produce. Fabulous!!! Bravo!!! and thank you for your unmatched kindness (no one has done it before at Billingsgate). Lynn also praised your kindness.

So sorry I missed you Brandi!!!

The best crop is your fresh organic love! Lynn

The Triangle of Life

June 24, 2013

Seems I should know something about the circle of life, but I am dealing very routinely with the triangle of life...use, reuse and recycle. This is a great venue for confessions, especially after I've repented :) I was dutifully driving to the recycling center in Pembroke until we got curbside pickup, which is awesome!! However, we were still disposing of garbage in used plastic bags. We have been diligently recycling anything that can go into the big green bin, but otherwise, not so good :(Now really is the time to kick into high gear reducing waste; food and plastic! I am, as you know, shopping ALL the time and needing to use those plastic produce bags, LOTS of them, YIKES! Also, I am creating about a gallon of food waste a DAY with my juicer. YIKES!

At work, we are always all about continuous process improvement. So every day, I get a little better. For two years, I worked at the Pembroke Farmers' Market selling eco-friendly products. I have a stockpile of just what I need. First, I have Produce Savers. These are little packets of minerals that absorb ethylene in the produce drawer. The second thing I have is Flip and Tumble mesh produce bags. This enables me to bring my own reusable bags to the store for my loose veggies and not use the ones the store provides. Unfortunately, leafy veggies seems to wilt much faster when I don't store them in a bag, so I use Biobags, which are compostable plastic bags, made of corn starch and are safe for food storage. I can use these over and over again. Now, I also have a garbage pail. Remember those? And when I am done prepping all my food for the day, I walk that garbage out into the woods where I am building a very large garbage pile! To say I am "composting" would be giving me too much credit.

Now, thinking ahead to the winter and a foot of snow on the ground, does anyone have blueprints for a catapult? I DO need an efficient way of getting the garbage into the woods.

Like Bill Withers said:

My friends feel it's their appointed duty
They keep trying to tell me all you want to do is REuse me
But my answer to all that "REuse me" stuff is...
I wanna spread the news that if it feels this good getting REused
Oh, you just keep on REusing me until you REuse me up
Until you REuse me up

Okay, maybe he didn't say it quite like that. I love that song! Know, for you, I'm here for the REusing!

Love, Lynn

Long Day

June 25, 2013

Whew! Long day...maybe trying to fit too much in. I was up at 6:00 wide awake. Did some stuff on the computer, had breakfast, went for my walk, went to Newton Wellesley Hospital for my second BCG appt. I stopped at work on the way home just to say hi to folks and deliver a thank you card to coworkers, went to vote. I lost my phone, retrieved my phone, met with cousin Lisa for a few minutes, met with Reagan, who sold me a Cutco knife, after we chopped up a dozen carrots, took a quick nap somewhere in there, missed supper :(went to church :)...did I mention, Whew?

The BCG treatment is working better this time around. I know because this TB stuff they put into my bladder is supposed to irritate the bladder. Well, as soon as my two hours of holding this in my bladder is up, then I have to go to the bathroom constantly for the next few hours and it really hurts to go, just as if I had a bladder infection. Never thought I'd be so excited about that!!!!

Will love you in my dreams! Love, Lynn

"Certified Organic"

June 26, 2013

I keep reading all kinds of horrible stuff about Montsano, the ag/chemical company that is taking over the world. They engineer seed to be resistant to Roundup, which they also make. See how this works? They sell the farmer the seed and then sell the farmer the Roundup, which is so toxic it should not even be allowed on the planet!! Yes, I do have some in my garage, I'm sad to say. I understand you can kill weeds with vinegar. I have not tried it yet. In Whole Foods, these genetically engineered foods are labelled as "natural," yeah, naturally messed with.

The point is if you really want to eat healthy food, it must be labeled, "certified organic." Even "organic" is no promise that it really is. Let me repeat, if you really want to eat healthy, toxin free food, it should be labeled, "certified organic." That's all.

Call me a purist, but I'm purely watching out for you, whom I love! Lynn

Full Disclosure

June 27, 2013

I have been hesitant to share the true cost of this Gerson therapy in all its glory because, prayerfully, this therapy will be a significant contributing factor to my complete healing and I will want to promote its effectiveness. The problem is the route I have taken is almost the most expensive way I could go, well...because I'm worth it!!! The average Jane or Joe will not have resources to go the route I have gone, but I also want people to know the truth. We need truth to make wise decisions and to plan ahead.

I think it was on April 21 that I woke with an epiphany that Gerson was the way to go and that I needed to pull out all the stops to save my bladder and more importantly my long term health. I'm not sure if I shared this with you before, but I will now and then I can talk about some short cuts.

$5000.00	The Longevity Center
$1000.00	Travel to the Longevity Center and hotel stay
$2400.00	Norwalk Juicer
$2500.00	Infrared sauna
$465.00	Water Distiller
$189.00	Air purifier for basement
$109.00	Air purifier for den
$375.00	First order of supplements
And	
$200.00	Average cost per week for 5 weeks for food and supplements

You can see that the initial cost was $12,000.00. Pretty hefty, yes! On the other hand, each time I am rolled into surgery for my bladder it is $15,000.00 or more. Obviously, it makes a difference when I don't have to pay. But, I am trying to save my life and people spend WAY more than this on a wedding day! The Longevity Center is one place for learning the therapy. There are others; some more expensive, some less expensive. However, I have heard lots of testimonies where people have read the book and learned on their own. If push comes to shove, that works. The Norwalk juicer is supposed to be the best on the planet. There are other ways to juice. The Champion juicer and a separate press will work as well. I could have saved maybe another $1000.00 to go that route. I could also buy distilled water at $1.35 a gallon at 2 or 3 gallons a day. I certainly didn't need to buy the sauna. That is not actually prescribed by Gerson. I just wanted to get that edge.

I pray that you never need Gerson, but I also pray that you save for a rainy day for whatever challenge comes your way. In the middle of crisis, you do NOT want finances to be an obstacle!!!

Love you when it rains and when it shines!!! Love, Lynn

He Makes Up the Difference

June 28, 2013

I probably shouldn't even be writing now, as I have had a super frustrating day with my home owners' insurance company. I filed a claim on 2/13. The checks finally came today, but I could not cash them because they have my old mortgage company listed on the checks. Of course it is my fault. Now everything has to go back and be all done over. It is days like this that remind me that this world is not where I put my hope. Here, we face obstacle after obstacle, challenge after challenge. And even though I prosper beyond the other 99%, ok 98%, of people everywhere, I still find plenty to complain about. I watched a great documentary last night about people who worked in the largest landfill in the world in Brazil. It is called, *Wasteland*. I was given a great perspective on the riches of my own life, but still, contentment with this world is so fleeting, is it not?

Psalm 103:13-18

As a father has compassion on his children,
*   so the Lord has compassion on those who fear him;*
for he knows how we are formed,
*   he remembers that we are dust.*
The life of mortals is like grass,
*   they flourish like a flower of the field;*
the wind blows over it and it is gone,
*   and its place remembers it no more.*
But from everlasting to everlasting
*   the Lord's love is with those who fear him,*
*   and his righteousness with their children's children—*
with those who keep his covenant
*   and remember to obey his precepts.*

Thank you God, for your everlasting love and patience with me.

Love, Lynn

One, Two Punch

June 30, 2013

Wow! Really rough few days! The Gerson book warns of two things happening during this therapy. First, it warns of the patient hitting a wall emotionally, maybe getting depressed or even lashing out toward those helping, maybe wanting to quit the therapy or getting really angry. I'm not sure I hit THAT wall, but I was in a really dark place for the past 3 days. This is probably common for all with illness. You saw a little of that in my Friday post. At first, I thought it was people, things wrong with the world, not me. Then I realized, things that I usually overlook are REALLY bothering me. There have been moments I have been on the verge of rage or melting into a pool of tears. I know something is wrong when I begin to lose self-control. We exercise self-control on 3 levels: what we think, what we say and what we do. What I say and what I do seem to still be intact for the most part, but what I think has all been shot to hell. I'm not in the habit of cursing, but lately profanity fills my head over the stupidest things. God, forgive me. Luckily, it hasn't spilled out of my mouth, yet. "Taking every thought captive for Christ," has not really been working. The second place we practice self-control is in what we say. I prayed that I wouldn't say anything hurtful to anyone at church today. Believe me, saying something insensitive is not hard for me to do. I was in a gathering of about 2500 to 3000 people today. The love and encouragement there was enough to sooth this simmering beast. The third level we practice self-control is what we do. I did not feel safe in my car today. At one point, I looked down and saw that I was traveling at 90 miles an hour. My head was just not in the game. I just was not paying attention.

Punch two: emotionally, I have been really off. The second thing the Gerson book warns of is "healing reactions." These are times when your body gets really sick for a short period on its way to complete healing. I think this usually comes in the form of fever and chills or some other immune response. I got REALLY ill today but don't think it was a "healing reaction." I started getting a headache when I was leaving church. I stopped at Mickey D's, (yes, way off) and got some fries on the way home. By the time I got home, the pain in my head was so bad, I vomited my fries. Not sure if it was pain induced vomiting or fast food induced vomiting. The Gerson protocol for any kind of pain is Aspirin, Niacin and vitamin C and a coffee enema. So that is what I did and then I went to sleep. When I woke, I could feel some of that, "woe is me" darkness had lifted. I just returned from the movies with good friends Steve and Joe. My headache is still with me, but I'm sure I will survive. Fellowship certainly helped lighten me up. I'll have nightmares about zombies for the next two decades but Steve and Joe's company was worth it!

I think tomorrow will be a better day! Please keep praying for me physically and emotionally. I need God and God knows how much! I NEED you and pray that God shows you how much :)

Need you and love you, Lynn

Freedom List

July 3, 2013

As I contemplate the 4th of July, I can appreciate the idea of freedom and independence. I keep thinking, "Boy, I wish I could work on my house, I wish I could work in the yard, I wish I could be doing my part at work" and on and on and on. So I don't think I want to create a bucket list, a list of things to do before I die, but rather a freedom list, a list of things I want to do when I am free from cancer, free from the Gerson regimen.

Okay, let's start...no, I don't want to jump out of a plane. If I were to put that on the list, it would have to be last, just in case. I'm not so interested in travelling. I don't want to just see a place. I want to BUILD a place!! When I was 19 I got my real estate license because I wanted to flip houses, before it was even called "flipping." My brothers offered me a place with them in construction. I should have taken it, instead of all that college. I did flip one house.

Now, I want to build a Gerson Therapy Learning Center, that is of course if I find myself to be cancer free in 8 weeks from now. Yeah, 2 acres, an absolutely Leed certified Gold building in Marshfield, big enough for 2 guests, their companions and living space for me. Then after building the perfect place of refuge, offering healing solutions to those desperate for answers. Yes, I would like that. I know this is premature, but I've never had a vocational calling. Maybe this it.

What's in your wallet? Oops, wrong question, what's on your freedom list? No really, what's on your freedom list?

...I'm free! I'm free! I'm free to love you!!! Lynn

Fist Full of Freedom

July 4, 2013 7:23pm

My friend Amelia, you know, California Amelia, lived in Saudi Arabia for 5 years. She could not leave her home unescorted by a male. Once she dressed as a boy so she could go horseback riding. She said she mistakenly left her house once with cross earrings and almost had them ripped out of her ears. She did not have a lot of freedom in Riyadh. Most of us have limitless freedom. It is humbling to think how I have used mine.

Galatians 5:13-14

You, my brothers and sisters, were called to be free. But do not use your freedom to indulge the flesh; rather, serve one another humbly in love. For the entire law is fulfilled in keeping this one command: Love your neighbor as yourself.

Hey neighbor! Freely I have been given to, freely I give...love, that is, Lynn

Moving Mountains

July 6, 2013

This morning at the end of our yoga practice, Emma, the instructor said that her instruction was inspired by Ganesha, the remover of obstacles.

Ganesha is one of the best-known and most widely worshipped deities in the Hindu pantheon. Although he is known by many other attributes, Ganesha's elephant head makes him particularly easy to identify. Ganesha is widely revered as the Remover of Obstacles. - Wikipedia

That got me to thinking about another mover of obstacles. Jesus says,

Matthew 17:20

Truly I tell you, if you have faith as small as a mustard seed, you can say to this mountain, 'Move from here to there,' and it will move. Nothing will be impossible for you.

This is a hard teaching. On one hand very encouraging, on the other extremely challenging. I cannot address this scripture as it is. My mind does not bend that far.

But, consider this: if you have faith as small as a mustard seed, you will look at a mountain and consider that it might just be possible to move it. And if you HAVE to move it, your mind, driven by that little seed, will begin to work and work and persist in that work, until you figure out how to move that mountain. If you have no faith, you will look at a mountain and think, not only can it not be moved, but even too hard to climb! You won't even consider the possibilities. Your mind will even shut out the discussion.

My mountain? Defeating cancer. Believe me, this is like moving a mountain, with me and a shovel, but that is okay. If I must move the mountain one shovel (or one juice) at a time, then that is how I will move this mountain. And perhaps you have a mountain of your own. Chances are there is a way to move it!

If you want to see a mind blowing story, watch a documentary about the building of the Panama Canal. That was some serious faith!

Willing to move mountains for you! Love, Lynn

New Carpet Toxins

July 7, 2013

I know that on Gerson therapy, I'm not supposed to put new carpet in the house, but on July 4th I bought two small area rugs, 5 x 8 each and put them in our breezeway. Immediately, once we rolled them out, I could smell the very strong fumes emitted by the rugs. I read that carpet fumes are just like any other poison and can give you symptoms other poisons can give you. I literally hold my breath now when I pass through this room. Luckily, I can open many doors to air out the room and can keep the door to the main house closed. New carpets can "out gas" for up to a year. Unfortunately, the toxic smell will probably go away before the carpet has finished out gassing and I will forget to hold my breath. The safe alternative for carpeting is pure wool, untreated, undyed. Yes, they cost more money and will last up to 50 years. If you are getting new carpet, consider purchasing at a time of the year when you can keep the windows and doors open.

Wishing I had a magic carpet to fly to you! Love, Lynn

Peace

July 10, 2013

The Apostle Paul addresses the Philippian church from a jail cell in Rome. He would never again be a free man.

Philippians 4:4-9

Rejoice in the Lord always. I will say it again: Rejoice! Let your gentleness be evident to all. The Lord is near. Do not be anxious about anything, but in every situation, by prayer and petition, with thanksgiving, present your requests to God. And the peace of God, which transcends all understanding, will guard your hearts and your minds in Christ Jesus.

Finally, brothers and sisters, whatever is true, whatever is noble, whatever is right, whatever is pure, whatever is lovely, whatever is admirable—if anything is excellent or praiseworthy—think about such things. Whatever you have learned or received or heard from me, or seen in me—put it into practice. And the God of peace will be with you.

All of us could read, "Rejoice in the Lord always" and stop right there. How can anyone rejoice ALWAYS? Is this not a place of suffering, challenge and hardship? But he goes on..." The Lord is near" and "by prayer and petition." Paul was in a horrible place! The absence of his loved ones was probably the toughest thing. But I bet the food was lousy too and he probably saw a few rats. So what was his secret? He had been on a long journey, but it was a journey he took, not only with God, but because of God. He had pursued God and now had the peace of God. And what is that peace that only God can give? The knowledge that we are not alone, ever; never have been, never will be, ever! That's a good starting place.

Lift your cup! To never being alone, ever! Love, Lynn

Essiac Cancer Cure

July 12, 2013

I sat down an hour and a half ago to write about Essiac, but got caught up on You Tube watching a documentary called, *Cancer: the Forbidden Cures.*

I love this movie because it shows how each doctor discovered a cure and ALL the people they cured and how the government comes down on them and crushes the good work they do. I don't love THAT. I love the stories being told, unburied for us to know!!

I just ordered Essiac pills prior to seeing the movie and now am even more confident that this herbal supplement will aid in my therapy. When I was in CA, a woman, Allie, came to see me. She had a brochure in hand and shared a story about a man she knows who has successfully reduced his tumors with Essiac. I'm open. I'm in.

Nighty, Night!! Sweet dreams, sweet ones! Love, Lynn

Swim Across America

July 15, 2013

I think I had heard of this fundraising event, but couldn't have told you what it was or what it was for. My friend Brian Smith swims every year for this event. This year he swam in my honor. Hey, that's very cool! He even had my picture on his fundraising page and a little blurb. So I was literally his poster child. He usually swims 1 mile in the ocean. However, it was so windy, event people did not allow anyone to go the mile distance. He went a half mile instead. He is no pup. I was at his 60th birthday party last summer. Bravo Brian! He even gave me his swim cap as a trophy of sorts! He was the 5th highest fundraiser. All donations will be going to Dana Farber for cancer research. Thanks Brian! You know how to make a girl feel special!!

Did you know that the phrase, "go the extra mile" comes from the Bible? There are a ton of sayings that do. Jesus said if someone asks you to walk a mile, go an extra mile. This was because a Roman soldier passing through town could ask any local to carry his stuff for a mile. Of course the Romans were the occupiers so no one wanted to carry anything for them. Disciples were to stand out by doing more than was asked of them.

Of course! I'll go the extra mile for you. Just don't ask me to swim it! Lots of love, Lynn

Honeybees in the Coal Mine

July 16, 2013

I know you think I go looking for this stuff and I know you think I am an alarmist, but I really wasn't looking, although at some point I did pick this movie. I received from Netflix a movie called, *Vanishing Bees*. When I got it I thought it was just a regular movie, but it was a documentary. We all know that the honeybees started vanishing years ago, right. Our veggies would be 10 times their price if we lost all our honey bees, if we even had veggies at all. Do you know the end of the story? What happened? Well, they started vanishing in the US in about 2002 or 2003. One guy, the largest bee keeper in the world lost 40 thousand hives, 2 BILLION bees in just a few weeks. It turns out that mostly the big commercial bee keepers were losing their bees. Devastating! Scientists were scrambling to figure it out. They found that the dead bees' immune systems were highly compromised and they had all kinds of disease, but they found out that France also suffered the same plight in 1994. It turned out that the SYSTEMIC pesticides from a German chemical company were killing the bees. That chemical company will not admit to that, but once the pesticides were banned the bees came back. Eventually, the EPA or somebody here in the states also banned the pesticides in the US and the bees came back.

There are some frightening truths. First the bees had already been compromised by commercial practices. Keepers were breeding and replacing Queen bees. They were also taking honey and feeding the bees sugar water. That's like taking mother's milk from a baby and replacing it with Mountain Dew. You see this? It is not just a slippery slope, but a cliff we always want to run to and jump off in the name of greed!

The really scary stuff of course has to do with a chemical company, a German company charged with the task of coming up with chemical warfare stuff for WW II, also a trusted aspirin company. So when the war ended and they had all these deadly chemicals created to kill people, they decided to make pesticides out of them and spray them on our plants!!!! Do you see the cliff yet? So some idiot decides how about instead of spraying on the plant we coat the seeds so the whole plant, inside and out, will be protected because the pesticide is now in every fiber of the plant!!! I'll stop there. We only banned the pesticide that was killing the bees. What else is going on inside our plants? ...I'm all organic! AND, when you buy honey, buy local honey. If you are paying $2.50 or $3.00 you are probably also getting sugar water from China or something worse. Buyer Beware!

LOL! My next movie is called, *Dirt*. This is the trailer:

Dirt takes center stage in this entertaining yet poignant documentary, which unearths our cosmic connection to soil and explores how diverse groups of people are uniting to save the natural resource.

Honey, BEE mine! Lots of Love, Lynn

115 Pound Weakling

July 18, 2013

I was very excited to hang my archery target on a huge Pine at the edge of the woods today. I got out my new equipment and strung my bow, with great difficulty however. I stood back from the target, loaded my bow and attempted to draw the string back to fire. WOW! I got a big surprise...NO upper body strength at all. Last summer I was shooting pretty well. My bow has a 35 lb. pull to it, which means it takes 35 pounds of pressure to draw back the string. I could only draw the string back about half way. Very disappointing. Well, I guess that's how it works. I stopped working out in November when my tumor was discovered. I've only walked and done yoga since then. This will be good for me. I'll just shoot a little, a couple times a week and then I should be up to par in no time. In the meantime, if you want to arm wrestle, NO!

Psalm 91:1-5

Whoever dwells in the shelter of the Most High
will rest in the shadow of the Almighty.
I will say of the Lord, "He is my refuge and my fortress,
my God, in whom I trust."
Surely he will save you
from the fowler's snare
and from the deadly pestilence.
He will cover you with his feathers,
and under his wings you will find refuge;
his faithfulness will be your shield and rampart.
You will not fear the terror of night,
nor the arrow that flies by day,

My archery instructor always said, "Fire at Will," but I could never see him! :)

Lots of love, Lynn

The Shoulders I Stand on...

July 19, 2013

Some time ago, Jan Stillings, the doc's wife in CA gave me info about a woman who had had bladder cancer and who opted for Gerson therapy. Yesterday I emailed her and asked her to share her story with me. This is the very encouraging story, so let me drop it like it's hot! She says:

Hi Lynn,

I just received your message. I had bladder cancer - they also called it "high grade" - 7 years ago. I had many tumors in my bladder, the largest one was 5cm in diameter. My Urologist told me right after the surgery that my bladder had to be removed. I was so shocked. Then I went to Stanford and asked the doctor who was the head of the Urology department for a second opinion. He looked at the x-rays and said that we could try BCG before taking the drastic measure of bladder removal. They wanted to make sure that they cut out all the tumors, and I had to have a second surgery. They didn't find any more tumors. I had 3 BCG treatments afterwards, but I felt this was not the way to go for me.

Then I found out about the Gerson Therapy and started it immediately after my second surgery. Friends, who had done the Gerson Therapy years before successfully, trained me on everything and helped me order all the produce needed.

I started with 5 coffee enemas/day for detoxification, and I had the 13 fresh juices, etc. I was on the Gerson Therapy for 2 years, and for the first 1 1/2 years I didn't even see a doctor, because their comments were not very helpful. They thought I was crazy. After 1 1/2 years into the G. Therapy I went to see a urologist for a cystoscopy, and it was negative, no recurrence (although they predicted something like a 90% chance of recurrence). I've had no recurrence ever since.

I am particularly encouraged because Christiane had the same "high grade" cancer I have and was told the same thing about having to remove her bladder. I'm grateful for her courage and thankful for her example. I want to be an example for the next friend with cancer or some other devastating disease.

YOU are my examples of friends in deed, in my hour of need! Lots of love!
Lynn

As Long as You Love Me...

July 20, 2013

Don't you feel this way: that no matter what is going on in life, as long as you have peeps, people who love you, that everything is okay? Even when things go wrong, terribly wrong, it's still okay as long as you have people who love you! There have been times when I was very alone, (I guess that's what happens when you're a loner). Even then, my relationship with God got me through. Over the years though, I certainly have acquired a taste for deep friendship and now depend on those relationships to sustain, with God, of course. So laugh if you will, but I love Justin Bieber's song, "As long as You Love Me", even the rap!! Here is just some of it:

As long as you love me
We could be starving
We could be homeless
We could be broke
As long as you love me
I'll be your platinum
I'll be your silver
I'll be your gold
So don't stress
Don't cry
We don't need no wings to fly
Just take my hand
I don't know if this makes sense but
Your my hallelujah
Give me a time and place
I'll rendezvous it
I'll fly to it
I'll meet you there
Now we on top of the world
Cuz that's just how we do
Used to tell me sky's the limit
Now the sky's our point of view

You're my hallelujah! Lots of love! Lynn

A Word from Down Under

July 21, 2013

My friend Emily form Sydney called tonight. She and her family are coming to visit for one short week and then they jet off. How fitting that she call right after I posted, *As Long as You Love Me*. She has loved me for a very long time!! I think we met in 1983. We were in a campus Bible study at Bridgewater State College (not University). Emily was so kind that I didn't trust her at first. I guess I just did not know many really nice people! I quickly learned that she was worthy of the greatest trust and she was a bubbling spring of the deepest, most loyal love. Even after all these years, she calls and she sends me little gifts from Sydney.

Let me tell you, sending gifts from Sydney is no small feat. She knew that I really loved the movie, *Australia*, so she sent me this really nice *Australia* leather journal. I visited Australia. I know how expensive EVERYTHING is. Most things are not made in Australia. Everything is imported. To send something to New England costs at least an arm and maybe a leg. And forget about instant gratification. I think it takes 3 or 4 months to get here.

That journal is very special to me, so special in fact, that I waited for a very special time to use it. She sent it for my birthday in 2010. My first entry is Nov 25, 2012, the day the doctor discovered the tumor in my bladder. The journal is chronicling my encounter with and victory over cancer! It holds all my notes from all my Joel Fuhrman videos, all my thoughts up until I started posting on Caring Bridge and it tracks all the weekly expenses of food and supplements.

Just her voice reminds me of God's love for me. There are so many people I would never know if it weren't for a Bible study group, wherever I've lived, over these many years. I only know them by the grace of God. I would not know them otherwise.

By God's grace, he has lavished his love on me, through ALL of you!

Lots of Love! Lynn

This New Body

July 22, 2013

It is taking some getting used to this new skeletal body! Most of my life, I've weighed an average of 140 or 145. 115 lbs is just weird. My bones are built for more weight so I have bones sticking out everywhere! Especially disheartening are my shoulder bones. I have always had a broad back. It has always been difficult to buy a shirt that fits. In order to fit my chest and shoulders there is always extra material in my waist. I knew I had bad posture, but now I really see. My shoulders are so rolled over they actually sit in front of my collar bone. I try to push them back, but they don't really want to go. I have to really strain to get my back and shoulders in line. Maybe I could wear a brace to fix that. Maybe it is too late. Also, if my shirt is fitted you can now see every bone in my chest. Speaking of chest, my bras hanging on the door knob are of course empty. They are also empty when I put them on. I went out and bought a few new ones today. I can use the old ones in the pool as flotation devices. Just being real :)

My bones are built for more weight and my skin is as well. If I could just take the excess skin from my upper arms and my thighs and use that to mold implants for the front and back of things, I would be looking pretty good! I have been perpetually shopping for clothes for 8 months now. I spent more money today as I am preparing to go back to work. Oops! I shouldn't have even said anything, because my co-workers will actually expect my clothes to fit, oh well! The shape of things isn't THE most important thing...at least for now :)

On the positive side...I do like my new face!

Facing tomorrow with you! More love to you today than yesterday! Lynn

Pave Paradise and Put up a Wendy's

July 24, 2013

Have you noticed, on route 53? They knocked down the last book store in my circle of travel, Walden's book store and they are building a Wendy's. Gee Golly Miss Molly! Do you think that is a telling sign of the direction we are traveling? I do. I know that most people just order their books on line or download onto their Nook or Kindle. But I have a theory…If you are a kid and you don't frequent a book store, I think you will be less inclined to want to read. Maybe kids get enough exposure at the library, but only a small percentage of moms take kids to the library. And we do not need MORE fast food!

Did you have to read, *Fahrenheit 451*, in school? That was the sci-fi book that has firemen burning all the books? They won't even have to. We are forfeiting them all on our own. When I was in school I only read classical literature. I am a very slow reader so I have to be selective about what I read. If I can watch it on the big screen, I won't read it. Since my school days, I usually only read nonfiction. Why not learn something if you are spending hours and hours reading? I guess many folks like to read for entertainment, but if I want entertainment I click on the TV.

A book I've been thinking about a lot is Dr. Seuss's, *Sneetches*. I had to look up the title. It's that book where a guy rolls into town with a machine to put a star on your belly. Then everyone rushes to get a star on their bellies. The point is, of course, you don't have to follow the crowd. In fact, if you follow the crowd, you usually just get taken for a ride. I think every child should have to read this book, then reread it as a teenager and then reread it at 25, 35, 45 and maybe by 55 we get the point. It is no wonder at all that Jesus called us sheep.

Love ewe and ewe and ewe! Lynn

Taking Stock

July 25, 2013

I just wrote down a huge list of all the things going wrong in my life right now and finished my entry on Caring Bridge and then mistakenly deleted the whole thing. I can't rewrite it all. The conclusion of the matter was that even with all the things that go wrong I still have awesome friends and family, I'm curing myself of cancer and I still have my bladder!

Habakkuk 3:17-18

Though the fig tree does not bud
and there are no grapes on the vines,
though the olive crop fails
and the fields produce no food,
though there are no sheep in the pen
and no cattle in the stalls,
yet I will rejoice in the Lord,
I will be joyful in God my Savior.

You ALWAYS help make things alright. Lots of love, Lynn

My Back to Work Strategy...

July 26, 2013

Okay, I have a huge confession....I bought another juicer....Don't look at me like that! It is all part of my back to work strategy. You see, the Norwalk (Rolls Royce) juicer IS still the best on the planet, but being the best takes a lot of time, too long! If I use the Norwalk, I would need 3 to 3 and one half hours of prep time before I leave for work. A couple people spoke to me in the last week about the new juicer on the market called the Fusion. It is inexpensive compared to most juicers that remove the fiber, $153.00 delivered with a 4 year warranty. It is very fast, at least twice as fast as the Norwalk. The down side is it creates more waste. I'm getting less juice for the same amount of food. But on days I work, the lost juice is worth the savings in time.

I timed my routine this morning. It's not all juicing. The coffee detox, we call that a "coffee break" in Gerson language, takes a full half hour, a 20 minute shower, about an hour to juice and drink 3 green drinks, cook and eat my oatmeal and juice 4 lbs of carrots and 4 apples. Another 30 minutes to dress and I should be out the door by 6:50 to get me in my seat by 7:30.

Okay, I realize you don't need all this info, but it helps ME to write all this down. My prep after work for the next day includes cooking a quart of coffee and straining it into a mason jar for use the next day. Then I have to make a salad for lunch since nothing in the cafe will be acceptable for my diet. I have to clean and cut my carrots and then package up all the ingredients I need for 3 individual green drinks. Oh yeah, and pack the supplements I need in a pill box for work. If I drink 3 drinks before work, I won't actually have to drink again until 11:00. That will help.

part three

The Honeymoon is Over

*Yesterday I was dozing off on the bathroom floor
or as I call it, 'the coffee lounge.'*

On July 29th, I had just finished about 3 months of Gerson therapy at home. I knew this was a tremendous privilege. I was covered by Short Term Disability insurance for the second time in the same year. Once my BCG treatments ended, it was time to return to work. I could have stayed out an additional month until I had my second biopsy surgery and maybe I should have, but I was eager to get this transition back to work over with and I was starting to feel just a little guilty about being out of work so long and feared the difficulty of acclimating the longer I was out of the office. My typical schedule for the three months that I had been home usually started at about 8:00 in the morning. Mom and I didn't finish with the juicer until about 2:00 each day. I would still spend time in the kitchen after 2:00, cooking something for dinner and taking my sweet time doing it.

Big changes had to be made to try to still do Gerson and go to work for a full 8 hours each day. I changed from using the Norwalk to using the Fusion. I timed all the tasks we did so that I would know what time I would need to rise in the morning so that I could get in an enema, 3 green drinks, breakfast and a shower before leaving for work. As usual, I didn't expect my Mom to rise with me. She was used to getting up at 8:00. I thought she would continue to do the same. God has blessed me tremendously. She got up and gets up still, at 4:45 with me. Because the green drinks NEED to be consumed within 20 minutes after juicing, I need to drink all three before I leave for work. If consumed too close together, they will wreak havoc on my belly. Therefore I give myself 45 minutes between each drink. I was drinking 2 green drinks before eating my oatmeal, but that was too much for my tummy. Now I drink 1, then have my oatmeal and drink the 2nd and 3rd. I take my carrot and apple juices and supplements to work with me. I keep the carrot and apple juices in separate Thermos' because if I mix them and let them sit, the mixed juices start to thicken. It is better to keep them apart until I am ready to drink.

I could possibly go to work early and then come home and juice my green drinks then. However, we like to use the juicer to do all the juicing needs for the day, all at once. Then Mom can clean the juicer just once a day. She is very particular about the cleaning of the juicer and takes a long time to do it. I wouldn't ask her to clean it twice in one day. There is also a great sense of accomplishment knowing that I have already consumed 3 drinks before I leave the house at 6:45 each morning.

I need a drink

July 29, 2013

My poor mother! All she hears all day is, "I need a drink." Now that I am back to work, I will decrease my drinks from 12 to 10, 3 of which will be green. Lots of questions about my green drink yesterday so here is the recipe. All the produce should be organic, but can't always find it:

Romaine, red leaf lettuce, endive, escarole, red cabbage, beet greens, Swiss chard, green pepper, watercress and an apple.

Now this is Dr. Gerson's drink with food that worked to cure his patients. He says, make no substitutes, but if you are of the mind to do so here are the top nutritious foods according to the ANDI score (the aggregate nutrient density index). These are in order of nutrient density.

Kale cooked
Mustard greens

Collard greens
Turnip greens
Watercress
Swiss chard
Bok Choy
Kale, raw
Napa cabbage
Spinach, cooked
Spinach raw
Arugula
Green leaf lettuce
Chicory
Romaine
Red leaf lettuce
Radishes
Brussels sprouts
Turnips
Carrots, cooked

Lettuce consider our options. Don't turnip your nose or bok at these! There are lots of choy'ses.

Love you lots, Lynn

No Greater Love

July 30, 2013

I was deciding whether to go to church tonight or not because of the time and my desire to get to bed earlier. I decided I should go and be encouraged by my friendships there and of course by our study in the Bible. The study was good. We had great discussion about many verses that we read. But it was at the end of the evening when I received the greatest lesson. One of my friends was asking me about my juicing routine and all that it involves.

Then she offered to come over for 40 minutes or so in the morning to help me prep my food for juicing. Wow! I thanked her and assured her that Mom and I could handle it.

Think about it! That really was very encouraging and very challenging too! I thought, whose house would I be willing to go to before my work day starts and give of my time and energy to help out a friend? I have no idea what she intended when she made that offer. Was she thinking she could come over once, once a week, more than once a week? She probably hadn't thought that far, but just saw the need and jumped in to help. I've always heard that a sermon is better seen than heard, any day of the week. And that was true for me tonight.

John 15:12-13

My command is this: Love each other as I have loved you. 13 Greater love has no one than this: to lay down one's life for one's friends.

You go first!! Only kidding! Lots of love, Lynn

Looking for the Bulls Eye

July 31, 2013

My archery target is neatly hanging on a tree at the yard's edge, as I noted earlier. I haven't been out to shoot since I hung it, but I see it through my window many times each day. It reminds me, "Stay on target, Lynn, stay on target." Well, what is my target? You have to be aiming at something, otherwise getting out of bed is really tough and now that time is limited in my day, focus is a new reality. These are what I am aiming for:

Staying spiritually vital:

Matthew 22:37-40

Jesus replied: "'Love the Lord your God with all your heart and with all your soul and with all your mind.' This is the first and greatest commandment. And the second is like it: 'Love your neighbor as yourself.' All the Law and the Prophets hang on these two commandments.

Staying physically whole and well:

2 Corinthians 7:1-3

Therefore, since we have these promises, dear friends, let us purify ourselves from everything that contaminates body and spirit, perfecting holiness out of reverence for God.

Staying on my game at work:

Colossians 3:23-24

Whatever you do, work at it with all your heart, as working for the Lord, not for human masters, since you know that you will receive an inheritance from the Lord as a reward. It is the Lord Christ you are serving.

Aiming for your hearts too! Lots of love, Lynn

An Ounce of Prevention

August 1, 2013

I was discussing the book of Proverbs with some friends tonight. The book of Proverbs is ALL about preventing problems. The word that kept sticking out to me was, "prudent." I am pretty sure that is where the word, "prude" comes from, which of course is derogatory, but I think the opposite of prudent is "wayward." Wayward is deliberately disobedient, unruly, ungovernable. Prudence brings prosperity and waywardness, destruction. It is so much easier to live life without our own man made problems. Life is hard enough. Like

Mama always said, "An ounce of prevention is worth a pound of cure." Here is the intro to the book of Proverbs:

The proverbs of Solomon son of David, king of Israel:
for gaining wisdom and instruction;
    for understanding words of insight;
for receiving instruction in prudent behavior,
    doing what is right and just and fair;
for giving prudence to those who are simple,
    knowledge and discretion to the young—
let the wise listen and add to their learning,
    and let the discerning get guidance—
for understanding proverbs and parables,
    the sayings and riddles of the wise.
The fear of the Lord is the beginning of knowledge,
    but fools despise wisdom and instruction.

Prudence, knowledge, discretion, understanding, guidance....I better keep reading...if I want to do right by you. Lots of love! Lynn

My First Week Complete

August 2, 2013

Well, I made it through my first week back to work. Super Mom has been getting up at 5:00 to help cut apples and juice carrots and rinse off my greens. After I leave for work, she breaks down the Fusion and scrubs it all clean for the next day.

There were a couple glitches this week. I had a little scare on Monday. I need to take supplements with me to work and I apparently picked up the wrong bottle of pills. I packed 3 niacin pills instead of 3 pancreatin. They look exactly alike. At lunch time I popped the 3 niacin tablets. Niacin is a vaso dialator. The niacin I take gives me a niacin "flush" making my face red as if I have been in the sun. Instead of 50 mg of niacin, I downed 150 mg of niacin. Not only did my face get red, but my entire torso and arms. It took about a half hour to go away. I didn't know if I might just explode right there. It passed without any bad side effects that I know of. I have been careful since. Niacin is vitamin B 3.

The other lesson learned: I cannot take salad to work. It is too much raw food. Ideally, I should have some raw food and some cooked food with each meal, but that is just too much work. However, my schedule requires that I drink at 12:00, then eat lunch and then drink at 1:00. Such a bellyache I had everyday around 2:00. I thought my tummy would adapt...mmmm no. Next week I'll take cooked potato and veggies for lunch and eat salad for dinner. That should help.

Did I mention this is the hardest thing I've ever done? Yes, the schedule is demanding, but really, it's the food that makes it so challenging. It is so tempting to feel sorry for myself. I have to constantly remind myself that I am majorly privileged and blessed to have the resources and the knowledge and the support to do this.

Loving you? The easiest thing I've ever done! Lots of love, Lynn

Which Way Home?

August 3, 2013

This afternoon I watched a documentary called, *Which Way Home?* It is about children who ride freight trains through Mexico, sometimes all the way from Central America, to cross into the U.S. These kids are in a tough place. They are either leaving to help support their mom who is in a bad place or they are leaving to get to their mom or dad who are already in the U.S. Sometimes, they have lost both parents and just looking for another life. Their hope is that if they can get to the U.S. someone will adopt them. They are children without a home in a very real way.

And of those who suffered for their faith before Christ...

Hebrews 11:13-16

All these people were still living by faith when they died. They did not receive the things promised; they only saw them and welcomed them from a distance, admitting that they were foreigners and strangers on earth. People who say such things show that they are looking for a country of their own. If they had been thinking of the country they had left, they would have had opportunity to return. Instead, they were longing for a better country—a heavenly one. Therefore God is not ashamed to be called their God, for he has prepared a city for them.

And Jesus says we too can get on the train and go to a better place, to a new home and a loving father...

John 14:1-4

Do not let your hearts be troubled. You believe in God; believe also in me. My Father's house has many rooms; if that were not so, would I have told you that I am going there to prepare a place for you? And if I go and prepare a place for you, I will come back and take you to be with me that you also may be where I am. You know the way to the place where I am going.

When you find yourself asking, "Is this all there is?" it is time to get on board. Come! Ride the rails with me! Lots of love, Lynn

Biopsy Surgery

August 4, 2013

Today is August 4th. My biopsy surgery is on Sept 4th. My 6 BCG treatments are finished. I imagine I am expected to idly wait 30 days for surgery.

Of all things,
I will NOT idly wait.
I will NOT fret in fear.
I will NOT sit on my hands.
I will NOT twiddle my thumbs.
I will NOT pace back and forth, up and down.

I WILL pray.
I WILL detox toxins.
I WILL move my muscles.
I WILL nourish my needy body.
I WILL sit and sweat in my sauna.
I WILL supplement with supplements.
I WILL drink my drinks, ingest my juice.
But above all things, I will NOT idly wait!!!!

...I'll gladly wait on you! Lots of love, Lynn

Lightening in a Jar

August 5, 2013

It is said that we are just jars of clay and most would agree that we are in many ways as weak and vulnerable. When Jesus stepped on the scene, he too came clothed in a clay jar. Yet, it is said of him, that not only is he the savior of mankind, but that through him all that is created was created and that through him all things hold together. His power is such that we will never really grasp it. His human form is merely a veil we can understand. In reality, he is lightening in a jar. Men often use the word, "meek" to describe Jesus. They confuse "meek" with "weak." Meek means, power under control. He has the power to set the universe in motion yet, as I noted earlier, Isaiah 42:3 says this of him and his mighty power:

A bruised reed he will not break, and a smoldering wick he will not snuff out.

I just LOVE this verse. If we are banged up, it does not mean we have lost the battle. If we barely have a spark left in us, he can carefully cup us in his hands and gently blow a breath on us to fan us into flame.

Come on, bring out the marsh mellows! Fire's gonna get hot! Lots and lots of love! XO Lynn

It's all Inside

August 6, 2013

Part of my "30 days to biopsy" plan involves taking something called Essiac. This is the name spelled backwards of the woman who first promoted this remedy in Canada, a way long time ago. She was given this remedy by local, native people. She was a nurse named Rene Cassie. Cassie had a free clinic that was curing people of cancer, treating 300 to 600 people a week until the authorities closed her down. Remember, if the medical industry cannot profit, then it is not allowed. She continued to treat people out of her home. She died in her 90s.

What's inside?

Burdock Root - Used traditionally to help reduce mucus, maintain a healthy gastrointestinal tract, stimulate a healthy immune response, for weak digestion, as a diuretic for water retention and to sweat out toxins through the skin. It has vitamin A and selenium to help reduce free radicals and its chromium content helps maintain normal blood sugar levels.

Slippery Elm Inner Bark - Contains large amounts of tannins and mucilages which are believed to help dissolve mucus deposits in tissue, glands and nerve channels. The inner bark, rich in calcium, magnesium and vitamins A, B, C, K, helps to nourish and soothe organs, tissues and mucus membranes and is helpful to the lungs. It also helps neutralize acids from occasional indigestion.

Sheep Sorrel - Used in traditional folk herbalism to cool the body, create sweating and detoxification through the skin: as a diuretic useful in maintaining a healthy kidney and urinary functions. It is rich in vitamins and trace minerals (ascorbic acid, mineral oxides, calcium, magnesium, phosphorus, potassium, silicon and rutin. It is thought to nourish the glandular system.

Indian Rhubarb Root - Used traditionally in small amounts, this herb acts as a gentle laxative and helps purge the liver of toxic buildup and waste. It helps neutralize acids due to indigestion. Its malic acid also carries oxygen to all parts of the body, aiding in healing and promoting a positive and balancing effect upon the whole digestive system.

I am taking this in pill form. Cassie I believe treated her patients with tea…no thanks.

Gerson therapy all by itself should work absolutely to cure cancer.

BCG treatment should work all by itself to cure cancer.

Essiac all by itself should work to cure cancer.

God, all by himself CAN cure cancer :)

Working hard, to stack the odds in favor of staying (whole) here with you!! Lots of love! Lynn

The Debt

August 7, 2013

I just got my Netflix movie today, *The Debt*. If you read the Old Testament you will see this amazing practice instituted by God among the Israelites. Every 7 years all debts were cancelled!! Can you imagine?? How fantastic would that be? And if someone withheld from the poor as the 7th year approached, he would count that as sin. He is always looking out for the little guy. Interestingly, he calls our sin, "debt." When we sin it is like we owe God.

Matthew 6:12

And forgive us our debts, as we also have forgiven our debtors.

Just as he was eager to see financial debts cancelled for the needy, he is also eager to see our spiritual and moral debts cancelled. But, did you catch the catch? It says to forgive as we forgive. Just 2 verses after this Matthew 6:14 and 15 says this,

For if you forgive other people when they sin against you, your heavenly Father will also forgive you. But if you do not forgive others their sins, your Father will not forgive your sins.

Yikes! ...But of course I have a favorite verse about debt:

Romans 13:8

Let no debt remain outstanding, except the continuing debt to love one another, for whoever loves others has fulfilled the law.

What can I say? I'm indebted to you! Lots of love!! Lynn

The Tipping Point

August 8, 2013

At first I thought, I will have to write about how there is nothing new under the sun because I didn't know what I would say to you today. But that made me think that there really is nothing new under the sun (well except that vision of technology by Corning. Have you seen it? Very impressive). There may not be anything new, but there are always new ways to use what we have and how we do things. Have you read that book, *The Tipping Point*, by Malcolm Gladwell? I love the book, love his look at the subject:

The tipping point is that magic moment when an idea, trend, or social behavior crosses a threshold, tips, and spreads like wildfire. Just as a single sick person can start an epidemic of the flu, so too can a small but precisely targeted push cause a fashion trend, the popularity of a new product, or a drop in the crime rate.

I was telling friends at the Longevity Center in CA that I believe with the internet, especially Facebook and other social media, that people will have more and more info at their disposal and I believe we will trend in better choices in the long run. Okay, people may still watch bad reality TV, but when it comes to important stuff, like health, food, medical care and treatment, the environment; I'm confident we can make better choices. Did you know that organic farming is growing at 20% a year! Chemically treated farms are called, "conventional." In the farming industry, fruits and vegetables are called, "specialty products." I can't wait for the tipping point to flip these terms around.

My heart tipped for you a long time ago. There is no going back! Lots of love!
Lynn

Freedom!!!

August 9, 2013

Now that I am back to work and every day is SO full, SO full, the idea of waiting till tomorrow to cut the carrots sounds like the best idea EVER! And the idea that I can sleep in tomorrow sounds like the best idea EVER! And the idea that I might be able to have a little down time tonight sounds like the best idea EVER!! WOW!!! I love it!!

...And the idea that God crossed our paths and hearts - the best idea EVER! Lots of love! Lynn

Crossing Over

August 10, 2013

We had the most interesting visitor today. Her name is Katie, a lovely and warm woman. She is the young wife of the funeral director, who took care of my father when he died. He will also be there to take care of my mother when she dies, providing she doesn't outlive him. Funeral home people used to creep me out a little, but this guy made everything so easy for my mom when my father died. And though Katie was here to see my mom, I knew it was right for me to meet her and talk to her. I embraced the idea that she would help me bury my mom someday. I think I was more open to this meeting because of the recent passing of our dog Lola and how Beth, the vet, made everything GREAT for Lola and us.

I see there is no reason to avoid those who will help me and my family cross over. More importantly, I embrace those who, for 30 years having been helping me, better know spiritually, how to cross over. There is no reason to avoid those who will help me cross over...

Romans 10:14-15

How, then, can they call on the one they have not believed in? And how can they believe in the one of whom they have not heard? And how can they hear without someone preaching to them?.. As it is written: "How beautiful are the feet of those who bring good news!"

YOU are good news to me! Lots of love! Lynn

Round and Round We Go

August, 11 2013

The problem with having to figure out stuff on your own is that you have to keep experimenting; trial and error, trial and error, until you finally get it right. We had a few conversations here about stainless steel cookware. I don't even remember where we landed. It should be magnetic? It should not be magnetic? One or the other indicates nickel and nickel is not good. I told you I got my new NuWave oven (as seen on TV) and the induction cook top. I bought the cook top because I make oatmeal every day and I cook coffee in a saucepan every day. Why not use a coffee machine? Just doing it the Gerson way. I find out today that the induction cook top will work only if the bottom of the pan is magnetic. The saute pan that came with the cook top obviously works. But, do you think I have one saucepan that has a magnetic bottom? You are absolutely correct. I do not. Lessons learned every day.

Okay, here is something that may be useful to you. The pan that came with the cook top is non-stick, but it is not Teflon which is BAD for you. This pan is coated with a ceramic coating that acts in the same way as Teflon does, but is supposed to be way safer for you. Induction cooking heats and cools faster and saves energy. I think it will be good to have.

I am not coated with Teflon or a ceramic coating. Sorry, sticking to you for the long haul. Love, Lynn

Not so Crazy

August 12, 2013

I know I keep sharing about Gerson, because Gerson therapy is my experiment and I am the lab rat. However, I have shared before about Joel Fuhrman and will continue to do so. If you watch Furhman and really hear what he is promoting, you will think, "No way! That's crazy! I can't eat like THAT." But trust me, read, *Healing the Gerson Way,* or watch a Gerson documentary and you will think, "Fuhrman? Not so Crazy" ...not crazy like Gerson. Fuhrman's suggestions are doable. They really are. Gerson therapy is of course doable, but only with really intense motivation.

Anyway, I have learned that illness is my greatest motivator or maybe wellness is my greatest motivator. I think the problem with most of us, is we get comfortable with the idea that having chronic medical conditions is normal and certainly manageable so, oh well, what are you gonna do? But take someone like me who has never been sick or had a medical condition and throw me into this cancer, medical, churning, grinding machine and I flip out. This is way not acceptable. I'll do almost ANYTHING to get well...except swallow down castor oil, no. Let's see, if my biopsy does not go well on Sept 4th, you might just see me jugging down castor oil - ooohhh YUCK!

Why am I going on today? We had an ice cream social today at work :(My friend in the cube next to me had a bowl of chocolate ice cream with M&Ms :(I didn't even have a bite. See, I will do almost anything to get well :)

Do you feel sorry for me now? Good, because I'll eat that right up!

Looking forward to ice cream with you, in May of 2015! Lots of love, Lynn

Many Advisors

August 13, 2013

My boss reminded me yesterday how much time passed before I actually found out that I had bladder cancer. In fact, it was at her prompting that I made an appointment with the urologist because my PCP failed to pursue answers. I completely trusted my PCP. She was my doctor for 15 years. Part of the problem was that she was my doctor for 15 years. I was her "Hot Fudge Sundae" because I always had a clean-as-a-whistle bill of health every visit. When I had symptoms of a UTI and tests came back negative, she did not test for cancer because I didn't fit the profile and had no contributing factors. My history had blinded her and my profile had blinded her. My faith in her blinded me.

My mom has said a million times, "Listen to your body." If your doc says there is no problem, but your body tells you otherwise, then listen. When your doc plays the odds with your body, push back and ask for the test. And if you feel like your doctor is not a real partner in keeping you healthy and especially if he or she is not listening to your concerns, then it is time to find a doctor who will be a real partner in your health and who will pay attention to your concerns. I loved my doctor, but I now have a new PCP.

Proverbs 15:22

Plans fail for lack of counsel, but with many advisers they succeed.

My chief counsel advised me concerning you. He said, "LOVE!" and love lots!
Lynn

100 Days!!!

August 14, 2013

It is hard to believe that today I celebrate 100 days on Gerson therapy. It feels like I just got back from CA, but I cannot tell you how grateful I am that 100 days are completed. I am not feeling victorious. I had no apples today, trouble in the market place. I am not eating the volume of food I probably should be. Having trouble getting down flax seed oil. Not always reaching my daily goals. I pray that Sept 4th will justify all the work I have been doing and give me the encouragement to stay calm and carry on!

On another note: I just wanted to take a minute to acknowledge and apologize for maybe not being there lately. Even though this page is all about me, I realize I am not the center of the universe and that you have stuff in your lives too! I admit and I'm sorry, if I haven't acknowledged important events in your life…a daughter's engagement party, a daughter's graduation, maybe the loss of a loved one, challenges at your work place. Maybe I haven't texted or emailed when you thought I might. Forgive me for missing a birthday, for showing up late and leaving early, for not delivering coffee on your extra-long work day. I'm sorry that you have had to do some of what I have always done, adding even more to your load. Sorry for declining the invitations to engage, to be together, to share together. My spirit is willing, but my flesh is put upon. My schedule is put upon. Sorry for any neglect you have been subjected to from me.

I love you! I appreciate you! I'm grateful for you! I respect the hard work you do! I need your great examples of faith! I need the love you so faithfully give to me. I don't tire of your attention or your precious affection. I thank God for you! Lynn

I AM and I WILL

August 15, 2013

Not to be confused with Will I Am, God named himself, "I AM." What we lack most in all of life is security. We want to know that if we fall that someone will be there to catch us. We want a home and a home base. The last thing we want is to be alone. God said, I AM to display his steadfast nature. He IS and always has been. He is not going anywhere. He is our solid rock. We need that. But I think because of our culture we can get tricked into thinking God is the big rock, static and passive, but there is another side of God that is dynamic! He desperately wants us to know that side.

In Ezekiel 34:11-16 in the Old Testament, God gets angry with the leaders of the people because they are self-serving and neglecting the needs of the people. God understands that we don't always have the people we need to care for us in the way that we NEED. Look at his heart on the matter. The analogy is the sheep are his people. Look how many times God says not I AM, but "I WILL".

For this is what the Sovereign Lord says: I myself will search for my sheep and look after them. As a shepherd looks after his scattered flock when he is with them, so will I look after my sheep. I will rescue them from all the places where they were scattered on a day of clouds and darkness. I will bring them out from the nations and gather them from the countries, and I will bring them into their own land. I will pasture them on the mountains of Israel, in the ravines and in all the settlements in the land. I will tend them in a good pasture, and the mountain heights of Israel will be their grazing land. There they will lie down in good grazing land, and there they will feed in a rich pasture on the mountains of Israel. I myself will tend my sheep and have them lie down, declares the Sovereign Lord. I will search for the lost and bring back the strays. I will bind up the injured and strengthen the weak, but the sleek and the strong I will destroy. I will shepherd the flock with justice.

God is dynamic and desires a dynamic relationship with us! Paul says this of God:

Acts 17:24-28

The God who made the world and everything in it is the Lord of heaven and earth and does not live in temples built by human hands. And he is not served by human hands, as if he needed anything. Rather, he himself gives everyone life and breath and everything else. From one man he made all the nations, that they should inhabit the whole earth; and he marked out their appointed times in history and the boundaries of their lands. God did this so that they would seek him and perhaps reach out for him and find him, though he is not far from any one of us. 'For in him we live and move and have our being.' As some of your own poets have said, 'We are his offspring.'

FYI, I think you're pretty dynamic yourself!! Lots of love!! Lynn

Life is HARD

August 16, 2013

Life is hard! I accept that life is hard. Accepting that life is hard helps me choose to be strong enough to overcome obstacles. If a soldier went into battle thinking war was easy, he wouldn't last long. The demands life makes on us are hard and I want to be ready to stand up to the challenge, every challenge and not just endure, but to overcome. When I accept that life is hard I can begin to correctly measure the cost of things I want in life. Once I can really appreciate the true cost, I can prepare to pay the price.

All my life I wanted to be thinner, in better shape. I wasn't willing to pay the cost. The demands are huge and call for challenging sacrifices.

Now, I want perfect health. I can't just take a pill. The cost is high. I am living and learning the demands, day and night and the sacrifices are challenging.

I want to be godly. LOL! I want to be godly in the sight of man and pleasing in the sight of God. The demands are huge and call for challenging sacrifices.

I want to build a home for myself and start a business for when I retire. The vision is ever so sweet, but the cost, yikes! I will have to continue to sacrifice and sacrifice and sacrifice in order to reach my goal.

Resolve, determination, perseverance, not wavering to the right or to the left, not caring about what the critics say, not letting someone pull me from my task. Life is hard, but when I do it right, all the rewards are worth it.

I Corinthians 9:24

Do you not know that in a race all the runners run, but only one gets the prize? Run in such a way as to get the prize.

No cost is too high for your enduring friendship and love! Lynn

Oh-Oh! Too Lo-Oh!

August 17, 2013

Well...I WAS 115 lbs. I weighed myself today. 107! I have to smile just a little bit. Can you imagine ever having to worry about not weighing enough?! Never ever thought I would see this day. Anyway, now I have this challenge. EAT MORE! I have to tell you, it really is not that easy. I went to Whole Foods today and ate about a pound and a half of food from their hot bar. Just wanted to nap after that. Tonight I baked some potatoes, but every time I went to eat one, it was not fully cooked. What's going on! Finally I ate half a baked potato and a big salad. I'm stuffed. Anyway, hard to eat what I am supposed to eat and get my weight up.

I had some blood work done for my Gerson Dr. My "BUN" was low and my "SGOT" was very high. The Gerson book says that my BUN would be low because of the Gerson diet. I have no idea about the SGOT. I emailed Dr. Stillings today. Hopefully he will get back to me soon. My body temp, which I hoped would go up over time has dipped to about 95.8 (skin temp) since I returned to work. I'm guessing because I am not getting as much rest, but that is just a guess.

When I was frustrated with my uncooked potato, I actually let the words into my head, "I can't do this." That is the first time. That is not actually bad for almost 3 and one half months. But I am really feeling my need for God's strength today.

Matthew 7:6-8

Ask and it will be given to you; seek and you will find; knock and the door will be opened to you. For everyone who asks receives; the one who seeks finds; and to the one who knocks, the door will be opened.

If YOU ask of ME, it will be given. Lots of love, Lynn

A Good Word from the Good Doctor

August 18, 2013

Dr. Stillings reviewed my lab work and had this to say, "Looks good. BUN is good to be low! SGOT is meaningless by itself. The other related enzymes - SGPT and alk phos are great. Keep up the good work."

Ahh, relieved! Otherwise, I had another plan. I heard the ice cream truck coming up the road this afternoon and thought, if I carjacked the ice cream truck and held the driver hostage, how much ice cream could I eat before I went out in a blaze of gunfire with the coppers? And of course another important detail I was thinking about was would I have to keep the truck moving to keep the freezers running? Anyway, now that I have affirmation from Dr. Stillings, I'll stick with the Gerson plan instead.

In the words of Sarah McLachlan, "Your love is better than ice cream" but I admit, some days, it is a close race, wink, wink. Scoops of love to you, served in a hug with a kiss on top, Lynn

Concerns for Vegans

August 19, 2013

From Dr. Joel Fuhrman taken from his website:

Legitimate Concerns for Vegans

There are some plausible reasons why a person might think that people should include some animal products in their diets. There are three weaknesses of a vegan diet: Plant foods contain no vitamin B12 (which all vegans should take). Some vegans have a need for more taurine (or other amino acids) and may not get optimal amounts with a vegan diet. A blood test can be checked to assure adequacy. Some vegans may not produce ideal levels of DHA fat from the conversion of short-chain omega-3 fats found in such foods as flax and walnuts. I advocate that people who do not eat fish should supplement with DHA or get a blood test to assure adequacy. These are three areas of potential deficiency on a vegan diet are easily remedied by taking supplements. Obviously, there are loads of advantages of a vegetarian diet that also should be considered, but that is not the topic for this article. A poorly designed vegetarian diet or one that is not supplemented properly with vitamin B12 and vitamin D (the sunshine vitamin) can be dangerous. However, these considerations cannot be used as an argument to justify dietary recommendations that include lots of high-saturated fat animal products.

I advocate a diet rich in micronutrients, especially antioxidants and phytochemicals, and the largest percentage of everyone's diet must be from unrefined plant foods-no matter what your genetic "type."

In order to do this, you must understand the nutrient density of all foods and eat more foods higher on the nutrient density scale. (Animal products are very low in nutrient density.) This nutrient per calorie density principle is what my book Eat to Live is about.

Fuhrman has found a strong link between a deficiency in DHA and Parkinson's disease, mostly in older men, but some women. Before I started Gerson therapy I was on Fuhrman's diet for 4 months. I have watched his DVD set and his stint on PBS, but have not read through his book, (small print!) His final plea on PBS was to just do at least this every day. This is NOT Gerson friendly. But if you are a fairly healthy person right now and do this, maybe you will never have to do Gerson.

1/2 to 1 cup of beans
3 servings of fruit (1 cup of berries)
1 oz total of nuts and seeds
    walnuts
    flax seed
    chia seed
    almonds
    hemp seeds
1 LARGE salad
2 servings of steamed green veggies
1/2 cup of onions (chopped BEFORE cooking)
and some mushrooms.

On Gerson, I now miss beans, mushrooms and nuts! Enjoy them while you can....and I will enjoy you while God allows. He is good to me! Love, Lynn

The Potter's Wheel

August 20, 2013

Jeremiah 18:6

Like clay in the hand of the potter, so are you in my hand

Have you ever used a potter's wheel? Surely you have seen a craftsman at the wheel or at least in a film like, *Ghost*. The first thing the potter does is slam the clay down on the wheel and then molding, spinning, molding...oops there is imperfection, hold everything. Mush it all back into a ball and start again. Okay, molding, shaping, spinning...until it is just as the potter designed. Perfect, right? Well, no. It has to be fired up to make the clay strong and if glazed, then beautiful.

Is that not our lives as well? Does not God continually push on us, allowing pressure from this angle or that? And does not that pressure mold us into a useful vessel? But not only that, he allows the heat to come, a heat that purifies, a heat that strengthens, a heat that beautifies.

Yet, if I don't allow God to work out the imperfections before the heat comes, I will surely crack and break when it does come. Therefore, I cannot be rigid and hard before he is done with me. I must be soft and mold-able beneath his fingers. When I give way to him, he is able to create exactly what he desires me to be. Feeling the push? Feeling the molding? Give way, like clay in his hands. He is the master potter.

Desiring strength in me for your benefit. Hoping you too are strengthened for my benefit. God Strong! Love, Lynn

Sleepy Head, Go to BED!!

August 21, 2013

I have always believed that you just can't break the rules and get away with it. Mom always said, "What goes around comes around"...and you can't hide anything because, "It will all come out in the wash!" Well, I've always broken the rules of good diet and I have learned that I can't, but I am quickly learning I can't break bed time rules either. Wow! I REALLY can't get away with anything. I set a new bedtime of 9:00. That gives me 7 and 3/4 hours of sleep. I have fudged on bedtime and I am paying. Yesterday I was dozing off on the bathroom floor or as I call it, "the coffee lounge." Today I felt really light headed in late afternoon. I took a nap from 5:00 to 6:00. Have got to try harder to hit the sack early or be sacked by the sandman.

Psalm 3:5

I lie down and sleep; I wake again, because the Lord sustains me.

Meet you in my dreams! Lots of love, Lynn

The Amazing Body

August 22, 2013

I imagine that some people curse their bodies as they lose health, probably when they lose functionality. I was very sad at the loss of my health, originally. It has been about 9 months since I got my diagnosis and I am more grateful and more amazed at my body today than ever before, not because it is MY body and not because of anything I have done. I am simply amazed at the amazing machine it really is because of God's design. I have lost almost a 3rd of my body weight (my body had plenty of fuel in storage). It knew exactly where to take that stored fuel from. I still have all my toes and fingers. Prayerfully, my brain is still fully intact. It didn't take all the fuel from just my right leg or all the fuel just from my belly. My body has sculpted itself just as it should be using only a fork, a knife and a spoon. Here is something I just found on line, posted by Brent Lambert (is he the Calvin Klein model???) Anyway, not scientific, but crazy fascinating:

The human body is an incredible machine. Part of what makes it so impressive (apart from the concept of consciousness and self-awareness) is its ability to regenerate itself. Your outer layer of skin, the epidermis replaces itself every 35 days. You are given a new liver every six weeks (a human liver can regenerate itself completely even if as little as 25% remains of it). Your stomach lining replaces itself every 4 days, and the stomach cells that come into contact with digesting food are replaced every 5 minutes. Our entire skeletal structures are regenerated every 3 months. Your entire brain replaces itself every two months. And the entire human body, right down to the last atom, is replaced every 5-7 years.

So get this, we look like we are aging, but our new cells just carry the memories of their parents. That's why even though I got this scar under my lip when I was 3 or 5, it still appears today!!

Psalm 139:13-14

...you created my inmost being;
you knit me together in my mother's womb.

I praise you because I am fearfully and wonderfully made;
your works are wonderful, I know that full well.

And you are fearfully made and wonderful!!! Lots of love, Lynn

The Bread of Life

August 23, 2013

On Gerson therapy, I am called to deny myself a boat load of different foods. I am really not supposed to have any bread except a special kind of rye bread that I am supposed to order from a particular Gerson supplier.

However, as part of my Christian walk, Jesus calls me to remember him by taking the "Lord's supper," commonly known as "communion." He says to break and eat the bread and drink the wine in remembrance of him. Different churches practice this in different ways. In one church, members may "celebrate" communion once a month, in another church, maybe once a week. In some churches, maybe only the bread is given, in others, both the bread and wine or in the case of my congregation, juice.

I do not deny myself this simple ceremony. I do not deny myself this tiny piece of bread. We are fortunate to sometimes have our bread homemade. In the tray that passes by are little round pieces, the texture of pie crust, the size of a Ritz cracker. Custom dictates that I just break off a very small piece between my thumb and forefinger and pass the tray. It is the sweetest bite of the week.

John 6:35, 47-51

Then Jesus declared, "I am the bread of life. Whoever comes to me will never go hungry, and whoever believes in me will never be thirsty… Very truly I tell you, the one who believes has eternal life. I am the bread of life. Your ancestors ate the manna in the wilderness, yet they died. But here is the bread that comes down from heaven, which anyone may eat and not die.

I am the living bread that came down from heaven. Whoever eats this bread will live forever. This bread is my flesh, which I will give for the life of the world."

These words caused quite a stir. His audience was confused and critical, thinking that Jesus was promoting cannibalism and in fact many believed incorrectly that the early Christians practiced cannibalism because communion was often taken behind closed doors. Well, Jesus was also described in the book of John as the Word. He was the Word of God in the flesh, but the Word for us today is manifested as the Bible, the Word of God. So it makes a little more sense if we talk about eating and drinking the Word. Regardless of the confusion, I love the bold promise:

I am the bread of life. Whoever comes to me will never go hungry, and whoever believes in me will never be thirsty.

It is a bold promise indeed.

LOVE communing with God and LOVE communing with you! Lynn

Time is of the Essence

August 24, 2013

When I have no goal in mind, time is plentiful. I have all the time in the world to spend any ole' way I like. But when I have a goal or many goals, all of time seems to slip through my fingers. Right now, I have many goals, short term and long. And the reality is, I have another birthday right around the corner. 52? Yikes! Time is flying. And in addition to reaching and striving for a goal, I have to do all that other ever so meaningless stuff, like pay bills, go to work, shower, eat, shop, clean, juice, juice and juice! Well, juicing isn't meaningless, but you know what I mean.

I had a French teacher my freshman year of high school who said, "If you want to learn something or accomplish something, you can do it if you are willing to spend 15 minutes a day on it." (I guess I didn't want to learn

French.) I have never forgotten that. Okay, where can I create more time in my day? I'm maxed out. Would you believe? I cancelled my Netflix subscription. Yup, both the streaming AND the delivery service. That is buying me a little time. And I just don't go out much right now. I don't have time! I used to work on my house in Wareham ALL the time. I haven't been to the house since February and there has been construction going on all this time and is still in progress. Not being there buys me a little time. I used to work in the yard here, all the time. I haven't as much watered a plant. That buys me time. The truth is, whatever I WANT to do, I CAN find the time. Where there is a will there definitely is a way. Most any goal worth reaching will of course demand sacrifice one way or another.

When something is important to me, even though it is not urgent and everything else is, I can find at least 15 minutes a day. How about you? "Someday" NEVER comes unless YOU make "someday" today.

Working harder this very day to make a better tomorrow for us all. Love, Lynn

Foibles

August 25, 2013

Isn't it ironic that when we are very young we think that someday I will know everything and I will be able to DO everything that I need to do and it will be just right? I am still learning that THAT day never comes. Whether you are doing Gerson therapy or you are raising children or you are trying to get a business off the ground, every day is a day of trial and error, slips and falls, toils and foibles.

My mom is half my Gerson operation. I don't want to say I couldn't do this without her, but I would be suffering greatly without her help. One day I walked into the kitchen and there was coffee ALL over the counter top and on the floor. It was one quart of coffee to be exact. My mom had poured the coffee from a pan on the stove into a mason jar, filling it to the top. When she lifted it up, the bottom fell out. The coffee wasn't even hot. That is not supposed to happen with mason jars.

I assume that with each week that passes, I will be getting better and better at getting all that I need to get done, done. This week, that did not happen. I forgot, 2 days in a row, to food shop, leaving me with poor food choices. Two days in a row, I missed 1 of my 3 coffee enemas. That is not supposed to happen.

Every one of us has lives filled to the brim with starts and stops, mishaps and foibles; and above all lots and lots of, "not supposed tos." You are not alone. We all fill the room together.

It's no foible to be blessed with your friendship. If I had no other, you alone are proof of God's love for me. Love, Lynn

He Reaches Down

August 26, 2013

For some time I have been thinking about a scripture and its whereabouts has eluded me completely. Someone at church or maybe Bible study was rattling off different scriptures and attributes of God in each of the verses. And I heard him say it, "In Psalm 18, the writer says that God reaches down to take hold of us." And I thought, that's it! That is the scripture that has been escaping me.

I went to Psalm 18 and read it tonight. It uses VERY powerful language to describe God's anger when he sees us hurting and I won't quote the whole thing, but it simply states in one line, "He parted the heavens and came down." To me that is profound. Of course, in Jesus, he DID come down.

Psalm 18:16-19

He reached down from on high and took hold of me;
    he drew me out of deep waters.
He rescued me from my powerful enemy,
    from my foes, who were too strong for me.
They confronted me in the day of my disaster,

> *but the Lord was my support.*
> *He brought me out into a spacious place;*
> > *he rescued me because he delighted in me.*

This psalm is filled to overflowing with the promises of God, yet, the reality is, is it not, that WE are often the eyes of God, the hands of God, the feet that rush in on behalf of God's good will and his deep desire for our safety, security, our peace? Is it not God's desire that we should supply his provision?

This world is full of hurt and want and need. Am I being the vehicle that God can use to wipe a tear, share a burden, supply a need, be it emotional or physical? Am I supplying his provision? What is that? Provision? It is one of those lovely words that encompass ALL that God desires to give us. Provision! It is deep and wide and high as the heavens. It is thick and meaty and tangible. It can fill us with inexpressible joy…And all of that can flow through each of us to one another. Challenging!! And ever so promising!!

Willing to face the challenges for the ever so promises of your partnership! Love, Lynn

Risky Business

August 27, 2013

My boss offered me a book to read, *The Power of Risk*. I would tell you all about it, but it has been on my shelf unopened for about a year. My friend Emily once gave me a picture with a caption that says, "A ship in harbor is safe, but that is not what ships are for." She is adventurous and a risk taker. After all, she ended up in Sydney from Lincoln Ma, or thereabouts. Yup, I'm still here in Pembroke, living in the same house the Fords have lived in for 80 years.

But, I've realized, you don't have to move to distant lands to take a risk. You don't have to gamble your money away to take a risk. Sometimes the greatest risks we take are just in the relationships around us. Kids are on their way back to school, maybe a new school with new kids. How frightening is that! That anxiety is not about, can I pass algebra? Ok, maybe it is, but more likely it is about, how do I navigate these new relationships? How do I know who to give my heart to? Should I reach out to anyone at all?

When I was growing up, I was pretty guarded. I really didn't have many friends outside my immediate neighborhood, except when I went to camp in the summer. "Loner" was the appropriate label. It wasn't until I got to college that I was open to taking a risk, letting people know me and trying to get to know people. The world is full of fantastic people. I regret taking so long to discover them. Because I didn't have a lot of friends for so long, I feel like I REALLY appreciate the friends I have. I've experienced so much more life and so much more love because I have been willing to take a risk and explore the possibility of friendship. And then, the tricky part is not drawing a line and saying, okay, this is it. I'm just going to stay in my own little circle now. I don't need any more friends. Every friendship is different and richly blesses in different ways. Why ever limit that!?

So glad you took a risk with me and I with you! Lots of love, Lynn

Hummingbirds' Flight

August 28, 2013

I am very sad about my lovely hummingbirds' departure. There is a long lived trumpet vine outside my window and I have really enjoyed looking out any time of the day and watching the feeding of the hummingbirds. Not only are they vegetarian like me, they also juice! They are colorful and delicate and miraculous in their treading of air the way we tread water. All the blossoms have fallen and my summer visitors have taken flight. One day as I was watching, the hummingbird darted right up in front of my window and chirped at me, as if to say, "Wanna come out and play?" It was like out of Disney's, *Enchanted*.

From scarlet to powdered gold,
to blazing yellow,

to the rare
ashen emerald,
to the orange and black velvet
of your shimmering corselet,
out to the tip
that like
an amber thorn
begins you,
small, superlative being,
you are a miracle,
and you blaze

From, *Ode to the Hummingbird* by Pablo Neruda

Genesis 1:20

And God said, "Let the water teem with living creatures, and let birds fly above the earth across the vault of the sky."

Superlative Beings, you are a miracle to me, and you blaze! Lots of love, Lynn

If I Could

August 29, 2013

There is a really beautiful song titled, "If I Could." I'm pretty sure it is a mom singing to her child, but let me just say, if you had a tough day today or you have one tomorrow, if I could

I'd give you 99 red balloons or
99 Gerber Daisies or
99 kisses on your forehead.
If I could, I'd give you 99 tokens to your favorite game
or 99 movie tickets (if I can go too!)

or 99 squares of dark chocolate.
I'd give you 99 amazing sunsets or sunrises, your choice.
If I could, I'd give you 99 pieces of Bazooka Joe or
99 lovin' spoonfuls of mac and cheese.
If I could, I'd do all the yucky stuff you have to do (well, maybe not)
still, If I could, I'd take all the tough out of your day.

Matthew 23:37

... *how often I have longed to gather your children together, as a hen gathers her chicks under her wings* - Jesus

Oh yeah, 99 prayers up to heaven for you! Lots of love, Lynn

Would You Pray for Me, 1, 2 3?

August 30, 2013

Okay, yesterday was all about you and today is all about ME, ME, ME! There is a children's song that goes like this:

1,2,3, Jesus loves me
1,2 he loves you too!
3 and 4 he loves you more
more than you've ever been loved before...

Okay, you know I have biopsy surgery on Sept 4th, so I'm just asking for a prayer on Sept 1, Sept 2 and Sept 3. The last biopsy surgery I had was on April 9th. I didn't even give it much thought or attention. I fully expected for the doc to say, "Everything went swell! The cancer is all gone. You are healed, you are free." Instead, he said, "The treatment failed completely. The cancer has come back and in many places inside your bladder. You have two weeks before we need to take your bladder out." That was his Plan A. Well, I opted for Plan B, another round of BCG and Gerson therapy. This time I have given lots of thought and lots of attention. My expectation is great improvement, meaning little to no cancer. My hope and prayer is COMPLETE AND ABSOLUTE HEALING as if I never had cancer.

Now a friend made an excellent point. He said even if the BCG doesn't work completely and the Gerson is working, there is nothing to say that Gerson will heal completely in 4 months, which is how long I have been doing it. Sometimes, its 6 months or 12 months or 18 months. Regardless of the outcome, as far as I can see, I will continue Gerson for a total of 24 months, but it sure would be GREAT if I could get a, "You are completely and absolutely healed." ...so if you start tomorrow, you still have one day to forget!

Luke 11:2-8

He said to them, "When you pray, say:
Father, hallowed be your name,
your kingdom come.
Give us each day our daily bread.
Forgive us our sins,
for we also forgive everyone who sins against us.
And lead us not into temptation."

Then Jesus said to them, "Suppose you have a friend, and you go to him at midnight and say, 'Friend, lend me three loaves of bread; a friend of mine on a journey has come to me, and I have no food to offer him.' And suppose the one inside answers, 'Don't bother me. The door is already locked, and my children and I are in bed. I can't get up and give you anything.' I tell you, even though he will not get up and give you the bread because of friendship, yet because of your shameless audacity he will surely get up and give you as much as you need.

Come on now, counting on your shameless audacity...shamelessly loving you and how! Lynn

One More Thing...

August 31, 2013

Could I be even more audacious and ask that before you utter my name in prayer that you consider saying a prayer for those suffering in Syria today and all people everywhere who are suffering: under oppression and brutality, from hunger or illness, from physical or mental abuse, from hopelessness or emotional despair. I am reminded of that picture seared into my mind of the Kurdish mom and her baby all bundled in blue, frozen in death, on a street in Iraq somewhere. Frozen, in death and hatred, all because of where on earth they were born. I hope I never forget that picture.

You are frozen in my love. Only my heart is melting. Lots of love and enjoy your fabulous weekend! Lynn

I See Dead Food

September 1, 2013

Who didn't like, *The Sixth Sense* and that forever famous line, "I see dead people?" Well, I'm not there yet, but everywhere I look, I see dead food. I ran out of potatoes last night so I didn't have anything to take to work for lunch today. That means my only choice was dead food. Worse yet, poisoned food. In Michael Pollan's book, *In Defense of Food*, his bottom line is, "Eat food and not a lot of it." He is suggesting that what we typically eat is not food, at least not real food. And how true is that!

Lol! At least the scriptures are filled with real food.

Matthew 4:4

Jesus answered, "It is written: 'Man shall not live on bread alone, but on every word that comes from the mouth of God.'"

You ALWAYS fill me up and sustain me! Love, Lynn

Generous on Every Occasion

September 2, 2013

I was thinking of a saying today, "Cast your bread on the water and after many days it will return to you." I never understood that, plus, I was thinking, is that really a saying? If I cast my bread on the water, won't I just get soggy bread? Anyway, it is a verse in Ecclesiastes 11:1. But here is a much more encouraging verse:

2 Corinthians 9:10-12

Now he who supplies seed to the sower and bread for food will also supply and increase your store of seed and will enlarge the harvest of your righteousness. You will be enriched in every way so that you can be generous on every occasion, and through us your generosity will result in thanksgiving to God.

There are many spiritual truths, spiritual laws that cannot be denied. One of my very favorites is that no matter how much I try, I cannot out give God. Not only can I not give to him more than he gives to me, but even if I try to give to others God will somehow make sure it still comes back to me.

2 Corinthians 9:6-8

Remember this: Whoever sows sparingly will also reap sparingly, and whoever sows generously will also reap generously...for God loves a cheerful giver. And God is able to bless you abundantly, so that in all things at all times, having all that you need, you will abound in every good work.

He also tells me in Matthew 10:8 *Freely you have received, freely give.*

I have received much and it seems the more I share, the greater the "much" becomes.

1 Thessalonians 2:8

..Because [I] loved you so much, [I was] delighted to share with you not only the gospel of God but [my life] as well.

Hoping to share all good things in every good way with you! Love, Lynn

Blowing out the Candle

September 3, 2013

With your prayers, I hope to blow out the candle lit in vigil, in the neighbors' window for me. It has been there a long time, since December. My hope is the breath of your prayers creates enough power to snuff it right out. As you pray for me, I will pray for others who are suffering. Thanks for your faith. Thanks for your love!

Biopsy surgery is at about 9:00 am at Newton Wellesley hospital. My sister Shelley is taking me and bringing me home. I'll keep you posted.

Revelation 8:4

The smoke of the incense, together with the prayers of God's people, went up before God from the angel's hand.

Revelation 5:8

... Each one had a harp and they were holding golden bowls full of incense, which ARE the prayers of God's people.

Lots of love! Lynn

Good News!!

September 4, 2013

Good News! The doc did not see any cancer during the biopsy surgery today, but still have to wait for biopsy results. He also said that a urine pap smear shows no indication of cancer. Thank you, thank you, thank you for your prayers. ...one more thing. I'm in a heap of pain. Please pray that I am relieved of this too!

I got home about 3:30. Have been trying to sleep and alleviate this pain. I have no catheter so I am in the bathroom every 20 minutes or so and still dizzy. I have a Scopolamine patch to help with nausea. There was something blocking my right ureter. I think something to do with a blood vessel. I have to go back next week to take out the stint he put in. Other than that, praise God for good news!

Psalm 13:6

I will sing the Lord's praise, for he has been good to me.

YOU have been good to me! Lots of love! Lynn

One Thing I ask

September 5, 2013

Sharing is caring! Today I spoke with a woman who had bladder cancer like me, but unlike me, was healed with one round of BCG treatments. However, of late she has been in and out of the hospital with all kinds of troubles and scares. I shared with her about Gerson therapy.

I was talking to another woman yesterday who has a really serious heart issue. She has been in and out of the hospital with severe pain and is on 4 different medications. I took her a copy of the, *Forks Over Knives* DVD this morning.

I got home to find an email asking me to call a woman I don't know, a friend of a friend, so I can share with her about Gerson therapy.

My sphere and my reach are super limited. SO, one thing I ask...if you are inspired by something I say and think a friend may benefit then by all means share it, on Facebook or in an email or on the phone or in a text or over coffee.

I believe only a very tiny percentage of all people who might benefit from Gerson therapy will ever actually try it, but I'm so grateful to God for my opportunity to know about it that I want as many others as possible to just have the choice, to just have the same choice that I had.

Thanks!! Even if you think Gerson therapy is whack, a friend in need may not.... Love you for putting up with my whack healing!! Lynn

Results are In!!!

September 6, 2013

My doctor called today to tell me the biopsy results are in and I'm all clean. No more cancer!!!! I marked the day on my calendar and realized Sept 6th also marks another significant day in the Ford family. Two years ago today my dad died here in this house of metastatic melanoma. I'm so grateful for the knowledge that helped me heal, knowledge we just did not have for my father. But it is knowledge I want to continue to share with others. I pray that God opens doors for me to do so. Just to clarify one more time with you:

One round of BCG "failed completely"

One round of BCG with 4 months of Gerson completely healed

I know it is called Gerson therapy, but Max Gerson didn't invent it, he just discovered what God had already perfectly designed. Food for health. Makes sense.

Much love, much love!! Lynn

part four

Living Victoriously!

"I see Him! Do you see Him?"

Of course, once the results were in, I felt vindicated, I felt victorious; I even felt proud of my accomplishment. I also felt that though I made hard choices and worked hard, that without God I would not have found my victory. I sincerely feel that if I didn't have 30 years of serious faith under my belt that I would have cowered to the doctors and done just what they said and I would have failed miserably. I don't think that I trusted in myself for this battle. I really feel it was the fact that I was able to entrust myself to God that made the difference in my path and brought about the excellent results I found myself with. The Bible says in I Corinthians 1:27 *But God chose the foolish things of the world to shame the wise; God chose the weak things of the world to shame the strong.* I think my experience with Gerson therapy proves this out. In this case, the "wise" doctors didn't have any faith in the simple, "foolish" principles of Gerson therapy, but of course Gerson therapy, in its God designed simplicity makes perfect sense and did the job. I have since seen my doctors and they still give no credence to Gerson therapy. I am solidly convinced in the amazing power of Gerson therapy.

Certainly, a huge weight was lifted from my shoulders, from my mind, and my soul. Prior to this victory, during the 4 months of Gerson therapy, of course I was always hoping, trying to be confident, but always aware of my imperfections in the application of the therapy. I could never really be sure it was working. There was no way I could know. The condemning words of my first urologist kept ringing in my head; "You don't have time. It won't work. The cancer is going to spread." It is common knowledge that cancer patients suffer from a constant state of the fight or flight response. When someone has been given a diagnosis of cancer, the mind panics and kicks into the fight or flight mode. The problem occurs when the cancer threat does not go away and the body does not know how to turn this response off. As calm and faithful as I tried to be, as trusting and rational as I worked to be, I know that there was a constant current of anxiety and trouble literally running through my veins. I often felt a rush of adrenaline rush to my feet. This happened as I lay in bed or sat in front of the TV or was at work, focused on a detailed project. I could not stop it, no matter what I did. Knowing that my body was producing an over load of adrenaline and probably cortisol too, created even more anxiety, because I knew that the excesses of these hormones was creating even more stress on my body. Knowing that the therapy had worked and the cancer was now gone took away all the seeds of doubt and enabled me to breathe a great sigh of relief and relax.

I reaped another tremendous blessing with my good news. Because I had been so very public with my diagnosis and my experiences, to be able to share my good news with all the many people who were praying for me and wishing me well at every step, brought me great joy! It is very difficult to share bad news. I felt like I was contributing hardship to friends and family. To be able to share that I was cancer free was like giving them a great gift, a great gift that would cancel out the hardship I had already brought upon them.

Moving forward with Gerson therapy at this point was easy. For the first time, I knew for sure that Gerson therapy is an effective treatment for cancer, at least for my cancer. I could drink up, knowing that with each sip I was reinforcing the good work already done in my body. I was also confident in the knowledge that, God forbid, if the cancer returned at any point, Gerson therapy was strong enough medicine to deal with it, until defeated. The all clear gave me more motivation, more determination, more incentive to move forward with the 2 year protocol for cancer patients. The challenge of course is not to get complacent as time passes by. My continued daily entries on Caring Bridge helped me be accountable for my daily actions. The correct execution of Gerson therapy is 1000 right choices. Then, to just make 1000 more. Then, repeat. The vigilance needed to stay on track is a steep demand, but so very worth my excellent health. I had to also make sure I was the one being vigilant. No one else would do it for me. Mom might reprimand me once in a while if I made a bad choice, but since Gerson therapy is so restrictive, it is really hard for people who love me to chastise me when I want a bite of something yummy.

Another thing happened at this point. Everyone around me soon stopped asking me how I was. The assumption, I think, on their part was that the cancer is gone, now everything goes back to normal. I still had to remind people that I had a full 2 years to do Gerson therapy and I told people often so that I would not run into resistance. I had to be careful to guard my schedule, which meant I had to be careful not to stay late at work, which had been my custom for many, many years. I had to make sure I didn't overdo socially so as to put my juicing schedule in danger and I had to continue to watch my bed time. I was really shooting for 8 hours and needed to keep that up even if it was an inconvenience to me and especially if I felt it was an inconvenience to others, who just wanted to spend some time. Luckily, my family and close friends understood the demands on my time and diet and were and still are super supportive. My boss has been watching out for me, reminding me when it is time to go home.

All of that said, the next several months of getting back into a groove at work and getting into a groove doing Gerson therapy, knowing I was cancer free helped me choose victorious thinking and therefore, victorious living.

Almost Normal

September 9, 2013

Hey, no comments from the peanut gallery about, "Almost Normal." Today went well. The doctor took out the stint. By having a stint in my ureter, the valve was not working. That is why I was having so much pain. Each time my bladder filled or I went to the bathroom, urine would shoot up into my kidney causing pain. Would have been nice to have a warning so I didn't think I had an infection or blockage. I had to have a stint because there was a papillary polyp blocking the entrance of my ureter, a polyp he cauterized. My bladder spasms which cause me the most grief are almost all gone. I still have some pain sitting in a chair or standing too long. Staying home another couple days to get it right.

The plan going forward looks like this: 2 years of BCG maintenance which is 3 months off, 3 weeks of BCG, a month off and a scope (peek inside) and repeat for two years. In addition, I will do my best to continue Gerson for another 20 months. THAT will be the biggest challenge. It is really hard to live without oil in my diet. I can only have flax seed oil, blah! But I will do my best. It was really good for me to see a testimony of a man who went off Gerson after 8 months and had his cancer come back. Good lesson for me. Maybe you don't want to read anymore. The crisis has been averted. My next apt isn't until Dec 2nd. But for me, I think I will keep writing. I think it will help me keep on track. It will help me be more accountable to myself and more mindful of how I am living and treating my body. You have been a great strength during a very difficult time! I am indebted to you and hope and pray that I can be as supportive and giving to you as you have been to me.

Much love! Lynn

Ready, Set, Go!

September 10, 2013

At different times along the way there have been very distinct, pivotal moments that have set my mind and heart in the right direction and given me a dose of drive and determination. Last night, I finally felt the victory that God has blessed me with, sink in. I felt revitalized, renewed and ready to move forward. Yes, I feel like I'm on cloud 9!

Today I ordered 3 copies of, *Healing the Gerson Way* and copies of my biopsy results and my urine pap smear. I will write a letter and enclose with the first biopsy results, the second biopsy results and a copy of the book and send to my old PCP, my first urologist and my new urologists. That is one thing I will do; not in any way whatsoever to say, I told you so, but in earnest hope that they awaken to the possibility this might help future patients of theirs.

And, where I have been growing weary of Gerson and almost feeling defeated by my cheating ways, I now feel ready to buck up and sit straighter in my saddle, get back in line and follow through with this thing the right way...okay, after a few celebratory meals. Ready to rock and roll, baby!

Psalm 91:14

"Because [s]he loves me," says the Lord, "I will rescue [her]; I will protect [her], for [s]he acknowledges my name."

And acknowledging that I couldn't do this without YOU! Lots of love, Lynn

Power Problems

September 11, 2013

Alrighty, I'm back on track. Did a full day of Gerson today and will return to work tomorrow. ...So, I was minding my own business and a funny thing happened. Our electric bill was $295.00 this past month. As my friends Emily and Amy would say, Grrrrrr!!!! Well, doing things the Gerson way uses lots of energy, but last month our bill was $200.00 and we think about $50 of that can be attributed to the pool pump. Thank God the pool is now closed. I'm thinking Gerson might push the bill to $150.00, but come on, $295.00 for 2 people???!!!

Here's the breakdown.

NO microwave.

Using the electric range about 3 times a day.

Using the toaster oven about twice a day.

Did use the sauna a lot right before surgery, but infrared is not supposed to use a lot of energy!

Oops! Every time I turned on the sauna, I also turned on the air purifier in the basement for about an hour and the ionic air purifier for about an hour.

Using tons of hot water for dish washing. (Mom, typically hyper frugal, for some reason likes to let the water run to overflowing and then some).

We are using 3, count'em, 3 refrigerators, OLD FRIDGES, like 20 years old each. (my brothers need SOME space for their beer)

We run a water distiller all day. It is basically a hot plate boiling water 9 hours a day. That uses a lot of electricity.

The problem with energy efficiency is you have to spend a lot of money to save money in the long run. Okay, we will see! Maybe I'll get one of those energy meters to find out where we are spending. Have to check on the energy use for the sauna and see if I can figure out if my "Power Saver," a box of capacitors that captures unused energy, is failing.

Powered by your love and support! Lots of love to you! Lynn

Celebration!!

September 12, 2013

Today was all about celebration. I returned to work today and though the news of my clean biopsy was already out, I just had to send an email to those who I knew have been rooting for me. It is a terrible thing to have to share bad news with people. It was glorious to be able to share great news with people. And I ALWAYS underestimate how invested people are in me. SO many folks wrote back, "tears of joy." Funny, I haven't shed any tears at all!! Someone wrote, "That is the best news ever" or "You made my day," "I will be smiling for days," "You don't know how happy I am for you." COOL!

Though I am focused on moving forward with even greater things, I certainly want to stop and celebrate this victory God has granted. Tonight, I met with friends Beti and Linda and celebrated! I still got home by 7:00, but we celebrated all the same! And I will continue to celebrate; special meals with special folks who have supported me and helped me through!

In the Old Testament God was serious about celebration. He is the ultimate party animal. And it wasn't dinner at, *Not Your Average Joe's*. It usually included a festival and 7 days of celebration. Of course Passover was the biggy, but there were a multitude of celebrations every year COMMANDED by God: The Festival of the Harvest, the Festival of Weeks, the Festival of Tabernacles and on and on. And as with all commands, came his promises.

Deuteronomy 16:15

For seven days celebrate the festival to the Lord your God at the place the Lord will choose. For the Lord your God will bless you in all your harvest and in all the work of your hands, and your joy will be complete. (How awesome is that!)

My joy IS complete in Him and in YOU! Lots of love, Lynn

Restoration

September 13, 2013

I have been working so hard to restore health to my body that my property in Wareham has been sort of waiting in the wings for me to give attention. If you remember, I had really serious water damage from frozen pipes during Nemo. Anyway, my brother Mark has been rebuilding the 6 damaged rooms. We are getting close to full restoration. I met with National Floors Direct tonight and picked out the perfect Berber carpeting to replace all the upstairs and staircase carpeting and at a great price. I prayed to God before the meeting to go ahead of me because I really do not like to negotiate prices (Dave Ramsey would not be proud of me). I was very happy with the price. After the carpet is down then we just have to replace the kitchen floor and the inside will be complete. Not sure if I will tackle anything on the outside.

The awesome thing about having your body wrecked by cancer or your house wrecked by a storm is that restoration can make either, way better than ever!!! I had health screenings today at work. All the numbers were the best they have ever been, naturally :) And I have NEW beautiful hardwood floors in my downstairs. Every room has been freshly painted. I will have new carpeting and new kitchen floors. I have a new body and I will have a house like brand new. Awesome!

Romans 8:28

And we know that in all things God works for the good of those who love him, who have been called according to his purpose.

Me and you? No restoration needed! Lots of love, Lynn

Great Plans!

September 15, 2013

When was the last time you were really excited about something? Two years ago when my Dad died of cancer, my brain got to thinking. My Dad had always been there for me when I needed help. When I realized I would have to live in the world without him, I started making plans to buy land in North Carolina so that I could move there when I retired. I was feeling the hostility of New England weather and just felt I didn't want to deal with that without my Dad around. I was very close to buying 10 acres right outside of Greensboro. Get this, 10 acres of gorgeous flat, dry land for $70,000. Right at the last minute, the deal fell through. I was going to have a truffle farm and the locals did not want any kind of farm on the property. There was no reasonable recourse. I was reconsidering my options. I looked at more land over the next month or so and did not find anything to my liking and felt like that was a sign from God, that he did not want me to move there.

Now that I have been given a new lease from my bladder cancer, I am all excited again about my future and plans I have for great things. For days, I have been designing a building that can house a Gerson therapy training facility and living quarters for me. I have a passion for energy efficient, highly functional and beautiful living space. How does post and beam strike you? I have been researching and I think it will be possible to build my vision. The very tricky factor, finding land along rte 3 for a price that works. And then of course, zoning and all that. Looking for at least 1 and a half acres, preferably 2 for under $250,000. Yikes! That is a tall order for these parts.

I am deadly serious about this and will be working every day to make this a reality for when I am able to retire from my job.

If I stay healthy!!!! I may have another 30 or so years of a second career!

Can't wait to give you the tour!!!! Lots of love, Lynn

An Everyday Discipline

September 16, 2013

You know, Gerson therapy is an everyday discipline. The every dayness of it was very difficult for me to adjust to mentally. I kept thinking I was going to get a day off; a Saturday, a holiday, a sick day, a vacation day...No go! There are no days off. I was taking my BCG days off, but I was running into problems, headaches as I recall. Dr. Stillings said not to miss any days. So now, I work hard to comply. I may modify, but every day I do Gerson to some extent. Now, if I think about taking a day off, it is like thinking about taking a day off from light. I can live without light, but I wouldn't want to go a whole day without it.

I told you that I would work every day to make my vision a reality. Transforming an idea in my head and then on paper, literally into concrete and wood, will have to be an everyday discipline. So the first thing is going public, which is what I have done by telling you. You have no idea what kind of power "going public" has. It is a very strong motivational force. If you know me, fortunately or unfortunately, you may have had to hear about more than one of my visions. One of these days, one of these visions just might stick and I'm planning on it being this one. So be prepared, I'm going to be talking up a storm!

Going public with my love for you! Lots of Love, Lynn

Seasonal Change, Seasonal Challenges

September 17, 2013

Today was the first day I really noticed it. When I got home from work, it was time to do a coffee enema. Just to explain, (cuz I know you are curious). I first insert about a cup of water and hold for a few minutes and release. Then, using my enema bucket again, I insert a cup of brewed organic coffee and lie down on the bathroom floor on my right side for 15 minutes, covering up with a bath towel. Then I evacuate a second time. On the bathroom floor, I have the bathroom rug, then a folded yoga mat on top of that and then a bath towel on top of that. My bare legs were on the exposed bathroom floor. Mmmm, kind of cold. The distilled water I used had been sitting in the bathroom in a mason jar. Ooh, kind of cold. The coffee, also sitting in a mason jar in the bathroom...yes, kind of cold. It is only Sept 17th. I think it will be an interesting winter as we strive to keep the electric and heating bills down.

Note to self: in the new Gerson facility, install radiant heating in the bathroom floors.

Note to self: in my new Gerson body, embrace the radiant you! Lots of love, Lynn

Do You See Him?

September 18, 2013

As I think about the events of my life over the last 9 months, I am amazed, more and more at how I see God in all that is happening. Often, I know that God is working in my life, but it isn't always that I see so clearly his hand and his love working so powerfully in the course of events. Have I told you the story? I mean, have I really told you the story? Look at how he orchestrated. The Bible never calls him "Maestro" but I think of God as orchestrating events, conversations, thoughts, happenings; all the time!

In July of 2012, I had never really worked out in my life, well, since high school. I happened to be sitting between two women at my pool one day, two women in great shape and super health conscious! That is all it took. I was struck with a very deep conviction that I needed to lose weight, start working out and change my diet. As is my custom, I went public with that conviction, telling Beti my resolve. She so generously offered to work out with me. What she really meant was, "Let me whip you into shape." For 4 months I trained with Beti, 3 times a week for an hour and a half each night!! I was working out so hard I asked my doctor for a stress test to make sure I didn't drop dead of a heart attack. In the meantime, I was trying to figure out why I kept having symptoms of a UTI. In addition, I was also doing hot power yoga with Beti's sister, Vivi. Vivi had invited me to try yoga with her. I had had many invitations to try yoga, but I always said no thanks. Vivi arrived at yoga class after working a very long day at the family restaurant. She was always exhausted and typically rolled out her mat and lay down, not saying much of anything. One night she came into class very excited about a documentary she had seen on Netflix. She said these two doctors claimed they could cure cancer and other disease without chemo or surgery or radiation, only food! Wow! That's interesting, I thought. In discussing my medical challenges with everyone who would listen, my boss and my good friend Beth said, "You need to see a urologist." A what? What's a urologist? Within two weeks I had my cancer diagnosis. Are you keeping up? So I run back to Vivi at yoga class and ask, "What was the name of that documentary?" Oh, *Forks Over Knives*. I watched and was amazed. That same week I caught Dr. Joel Fuhrman on PBS. Hey! He was saying the same thing as the *Forks Over*

Knives video!!! I changed my diet that weekend. Radically changed an already changed diet to no meat, no dairy, no junk food.

Okay, so I am doing the Fuhrman diet, I have surgery to remove all the cancer and I start BCG treatments. A full 5 months later, my urologist says, the treatment failed completely, the cancer is back even more so and will definitely breach my bladder wall unless we take the bladder out. During that 5 months, Netflix and Facebook friends kept recommending more food related documentaries. I was eating them up. I couldn't get enough. Time and time again, these documentaries kept pointing to Gerson therapy. I was intrigued. I bought the book and read the book. When the doctor said it was critical for me to remove my bladder within two weeks, God had prepared me. He had prepared me physically, he prepared me with knowledge and he prepared me emotionally, building my confidence. I said, "Have you ever heard of Gerson therapy?" He said, "No and regardless of what it is, you do not have time. You have a very small window."

...To be continued

Knowing FULL WELL that God has orchestrated you into my life. Of course! He loves me! Loving you, Lynn

Do you See Him? continued

September 19, 2013

My doctor asked me if I wanted a second opinion. Sure, of course. He wrote down a name and number of a doctor he wanted me to call. The next day, my mom called my dad's oncologist and got a name of a different doctor and made an appointment. When I called for a referral from my PCP's office, I was told that I couldn't see the doc that my Mom had chosen and I couldn't see the doc that my doc had chosen. Since I have always been healthy I have the least expensive health insurance my company offers. My plan does not allow me to see docs outside my network. My PCP's office suggested I see someone else. I was pretty sure he was going to give the same opinion as my urologist.

I was fearful because I was pretty sure I could go against the opinion of one doctor, but I wasn't sure I could go against the opinions of two doctors. By the grace of God, he said he would be willing to give BCG another try. This was the greatest news! This gave me the confidence and the opportunity to try Gerson and get medical leave insurance coverage while I was out of work at The Longevity Center and during the 3 months of BCG treatments. This was a great door opening for me. Who knows what the other two docs may have recommended. However, I will never know because God only left one open door for me to walk through.

And I am grateful that my 1st urologist did not say that he would give BCG a second try. If he had, I would have put my faith in that and not be pushed to try Gerson. I am convinced that had I given BCG a second try without Gerson, it would have failed just as the first round had. Then, who knows? Maybe at that point the cancer would have passed through the wall of the bladder. Gerson therapy works even if the cancer is spread everywhere, but I cannot testify with confidence that I would have been able to follow through with Gerson at that point. I would like to think so, but I just don't know. I believe that God took me to the brink of my faith and then worked out all the details. I can see how he used all kinds of people along the way, conversations, coincidences, etc.

That conviction at the poolside was like a tidal wave. I believe that was from God. I believe he sent Beti to train me, Vivi to inform me, Beth and Lyn and my mom to guide me, Netflix to educate me, Dr. Fuhrman to get me eating right until I could do Gerson, my first urologist to scare me into action, tough action, my second urologist to buy me time, Dr. Stillings and his wife Jan to demonstrate and teach me Gerson, Amelia, Janice, Bronwyn and Juanita in CA to give me spiritual strength and encouragement and friends at home supporting and loving me through every day! I see Him! Do you see him?

Romans 1:20

For since the creation of the world God's invisible qualities—his eternal power and divine nature—have been clearly seen, being understood from what has been made, so that people are without excuse.

As always, seeing his amazing love through you! Love, Lynn

Gerson Center Vision

September 22, 2013

I just have to tell you about one cool thing. I day dream about my Gerson therapy learning center and I've decided to name the bedroom suites, you know, like how hotels name rooms. One is called "Humming Bird", named for my summer time friends. One is called "Evergreen." That is sort of the masculine suite. One is called "Wildflower". I am considering naming my quarters as well. "Sanctuary" seems most fitting. I have one private guest room. I am kicking around a couple names, "Namaste" perhaps. Perhaps something else, something to compliment the color purple…Firefly? Butterfly?…hmmm. No, I have it! It will be called "Dragonfly."

Hoping you find your sanctuary, even if only in your mind, as chaos runs wild around you. LOVE! Lynn

Still Amazed!

September 26, 2013

I have been reading another Gerson book, *Healing Arthritis*, and thought, "Why bother, it is just going to say the same thing as the other Gerson book I read." However, reading actual case studies of folks healed of REALLY serious, "incurable" disease is absolutely fascinating and amazing. There are stories of people who couldn't even get out of bed and who the traditional doctors had no answers for. They do Gerson therapy for a time, sometimes short and sometimes long, but they are perfectly cured in the end!

Here is a list of diseases in this book, healed by Gerson therapy:

osteoarthritis, rheumatoid arthritis, lupus, fibromyalgia, myelofibrosis, scleraderma, ankylosing spondylitis, gout, osteoporosis, mixed collagen disease. And one just casually listed in a case study, CYSTIC FIBROSIS!!!

Here's one comment from the book about rheumatoid arthritis patients, "Cartilage reforms and fingers straighten out."!!!

Still Amazed! This is mind blowing stuff.

YOU are amazing, mind blowing stuff! Love! Love! Love! Lynn

Gerson Girl

October 5, 2013

Today, I launched my new Facebook page, "Gerson Girl." Within seconds of going live, a friend said she looked into Gerson and decided not to do it because she was informed that coffee enemas, done too frequently, could mess a person up. I think that there is plenty of information on the web that will support or not support whatever we choose to do. The info I post may or may not be correct, but everything I post will be knowledge as I understand it, emphasis on "AS I UNDERSTAND IT." As for me and coffee enemas, so far so good.

Learning, healing, growing, loving...with you!! Lynn

Energy Management

October 7, 2013

I was literally clapping with applause on route 53 on Sunday morning on my way to church. The wind turbine that has been idle forever was finally churning away. It was such a waste to have that energy creator just standing there doing absolutely nothing.

I was clapping my hands again today when Mom told me the electric bill was $130.00. That isn't that great for just 2 people, but last month, right before we shut down the pool, it was close to $300.00. I've made some changes that have definitely made an impact on the bill. Because I am doing Gerson and going to work every day, by 5:30 a.m. we have 4 appliances running in the kitchen. We start the "Waterwise" water distiller, a small oven, a cook top and my Fusion juicer. In early Sept we brought the water distiller into the kitchen. This little machine creates a lot of heat. I am hoping it will help with the cost of heating. I purchased a NuWave oven (as seen on TV). This oven bakes my potatoes in 50 minutes instead of 90 minutes in a toaster oven. I also have an induction cook top that I use for oatmeal and to cook coffee on. I just purchased an induction ready saucepan yesterday. This will reduce the electric bill further.

Gerson therapy is energy demanding! (on many different levels) but there is a lot of smart technology out there that can help us manage our energy costs. About 5 years ago, I was looking for a way to bring the bill down and found a "Power Saver." A power saver is literally a box of capacitors that hooks up to your circuit box in the basement. Every time you use an electric induction motor, meaning most household appliances, some electricity is lost. The measurement of the power you use is called a power factor. Most of us have a power factor of about 7 or so, or in other words we are using only 70% of the electricity we are paying for. The Power Saver captures that lost power and recycles it. You can reduce your monthly bill from 8 to 25% each and every month!!! It has certainly paid off.

So don't let your wind turbine stand idle. Manage your energy! You are gonna need it.

...You energize me!! Lots of love, Lynn

Building Strong

October 11, 2013

I was so excited to find a new book on the kitchen table when I arrived home from work. I am planning on building myself a home some day and decided a timber framed (or post and beam) is the way to go. My new book is all about post and beam construction. If I'm going to build something and I want it to last then I want to build strong. Hey, everybody is all "Boston Strong." For Boston to be strong then I have to be strong in what I choose to do.

Of course when building a home, I want it to last a LONG time. I don't want it to be vulnerable to outside forces. There cannot be cracks in the foundation or shoddy work, nor can I use cheap materials. Well, then, what about other areas of my life? How am I building? What about important relationships? I want to use the finest materials in my relationships: love, humility, forgiveness, understanding, compassion and sacrifice. Relationships will crumble to the ground if I don't use these things.

And what about my body? I understand what happens to my body when I try to build with cheap materials. It certainly isn't all about the outward appearance, the paint and the polish. Even going to the gym can't alone build a strong body. We focus so much on building strong muscles, but what about the rest of me? How can I build a strong brain, liver, lungs, bones, kidneys, blood, skin? I need to build with my fork and use the best materials I can find. My body, like a house is vulnerable to outside forces. A crack in the foundation can bring my whole house down.

1 Corinthians 3:11-13

For no one can lay any foundation other than the one already laid, which is Jesus Christ. If anyone builds on this foundation using gold, silver, costly stones, wood, hay or straw, their work will be shown for what it is, because the Day will bring it to light.

In this verse, "the Day" refers to the day we stand before God, but what we build with now will be tested now and we want to be strong now. So you can choose as you will. I am going to be looking for "gold, silver and costly stones" to build my relationships, my home AND my body.

I LOVE building with you!! Love to you! Lynn

Make No Bones About It

October 13, 2013

Let's talk about bone health. I make no bones about sharing info with you that will be contrary to your current understanding. Here are important things to know:

Our bodies are not designed to metabolize the amount of animal protein that we typically consume. In order to break down these proteins, the body will draw on our stores of calcium in our bones.

Drinking milk means drinking animal proteins, which means decreasing calcium stores rather than building strong bones.

Drugs prescribed for poor bone density cause more damage because bones want to naturally replace old bone with new strong bone. The drugs actually show a more dense bone, but in fact, the bones are much more brittle because the drugs prevent the body from getting rid of old bone. Women on these drugs actually end up having more falls, fractures and breaks than without the drugs. Some drugs have also been proven to cause jaw rot.

Calcium supplements are not helpful either because the calcium is not in a bioavailable state. In other words, the body cannot absorb the calcium in this unnatural state.

Just as an aside the milk protein Casein has been shown to be directly related to the incidence of cancer.

The best source of protein is from veggies, beans, nuts and grains.

The best source of calcium is in its natural state, from vegetables.

The best way to absorb the calcium we take is to assist with vitamin D.

The best way to keep bones strong is to exert a little pressure on them through exercise and getting enough calcium and vitamin D

Phosphoric acid which is found in most all soda leaches calcium from the bones.

Finally, I have some backbone to stand up to the myths. Truth, it does a body good!

Ezekiel 18:3-6

[God] asked me, "Son of man, can these bones live?" I said, "Sovereign Lord, you alone know." Then he said to me, "Prophesy to these bones and say to them, 'Dry bones, hear the word of the Lord! This is what the Sovereign Lord says to these bones: I will make breath enter you, and you will come to life. I will attach tendons to you and make flesh come upon you and cover you with skin; I will put breath in you, and you will come to life. Then you will know that I am the Lord.'"

I make no bones about my love for you! Lynn

The Harvest

October 14, 2013

I know that awhile back I talked about gleaning. Today being Columbus Day, I was just thinking of the harvest. I was just sharing with some friends about working on the cranberry bogs for my dad when I was growing up. Yes, he was a mechanic and a firefighter and a cranberry grower and a bar tender.... We had the bogs from when I was about 6 until I was about 17. When we water picked, which wasn't very often because it was a more expensive proposition than dry picking, it was a spectacular vision when the berries were afloat. Now everyone gets to see a glimpse of the harvest on the Ocean Spray commercials, which I think are fabulous. A harvest of any kind is a magical, wondrous time, but only the farmer knows the countless hours from sunup to sunset that go into the making of a successful, bountiful crop. And not long after the crop comes in does the farmer begin to plan and work for the next season's crop.

Thinking about my own harvest I have reaped, first on Fuhrman's diet and then on Gerson, I have to remind myself of the farmer. I took 5 months on Fuhrman (I mistakenly stated 4 the other day) and 4 months on Gerson to reap a cancer free body, a cause for great celebration. However, I can't just call it quits. I need to sow for another bountiful crop of good health for the next time I have a scope. I need to work for a good crop every 3 or 4 months. So, every day, I get up with the sun...before the sun rises and I work this soil till after the sun goes down. Only then, can I hope to have a great harvest every time I check my fields.

Hey, farming isn't easy, I know!!! But the farmer has invaluable lessons for each of us. Whatever it is you are growing, whatever it is you hope to harvest, till the terrain, sow in the soil, labor on the land and you will reap a great harvest! Whatever it is you are hoping to reap.

Even the words we sow with our mouths can reap a robust harvest:

Proverbs 18:20

From the fruit of their mouth a person's stomach is filled; with the harvest of their lips they are satisfied.

Sowing the seeds of friendship, reaping the fruit of love, with you! XO, Lynn

Stress!!!!

October 16, 2013

Stress! What a mess of your life it can make! Since I was diagnosed I have learned pretty well to live in a place in my head that is relatively unstressed. It took time off from work and lots of trying before I arrived there. But sometimes I just can't get there...I got to work at 7:30, at 9:00 I realized I had a meeting at 10:00 I hadn't prepared for. It took me 10 minutes to find the document I needed to review. I had to consult with 2 people just to feel confident walking into the meeting. At 12:00 I realized I had to attend a webinar at 1:00 on dealing with stress. Oh no! All this time away from my work is so stressful. I put my auto message on and "send calls" so I could focus on my "Less Stress" class, but as I sat at my computer I could see emails coming into my box. I kept leaving the webinar page to answer emails.

We are trying to aggressively attack some challenges at work so today there were 8 folks helping my team that don't usually help...8 people with tech problems, questions, needing direction. All great challenges to have since I have 8 additional folks! Before I took the webinar on decreasing my stress I could feel all the muscles in my shoulders tight, tight; my neck cracking and popping. And that tension just loves to creep up the back of my neck. After the webinar, I could feel all the muscles in my shoulders tight, tight; my neck cracking and popping. HA!

I know one thing! Stress will kill you if you let it. I need to step into work with a different mindset tomorrow. I need to have mindful prayer tonight before I close my eyes to sleep. I need to have a mindful prayer as I log on to my computer tomorrow. I need to accept what I can do and what I can't do, equally, with peace. One thing cancer has taught me: Punch the clock when it is time to go home and go home. I cannot recoup, recover, repair and re-energize if I am leaving the office late. Don't let stress kill you!!

I would not be surprised if I shared this scripture with you before. Some, we just need more than others:

Philippians 4:6-7

Do not be anxious about anything, but in every situation, by prayer and petition, with thanksgiving, present your requests to God. And the peace of God, which transcends all understanding, will guard your hearts and your minds in Christ Jesus.

Your love for me transcends all my understanding! Much love to you! Lynn

Stress? What Stress?

October 17, 2013

I took my own advice and prepared to go into work today with a positive and relaxed mindset. I was eager to set to work. I was patient. I was encouraging to my co-workers. I was able to deal with matters quickly and prayerfully didn't cause anyone else any stress. Some things got done. Some things didn't. Tomorrow, I will have an opportunity to do the same and day by day, we will make progress.

On Gerson therapy, it is really important for me not to stress to the point I am feeling great pressure. When I feel great pressure, I make really poor food choices and then I get angry with myself. There is a bucket of REALLY good premium Halloween candy just a couple desks away from me. I want to take it and throw it out the window. I have to walk by it 100 times a day, at least. Yesterday, I ate from that bowl. Today, I did not. Today, I am happy with myself. Yesterday, I was not.

I attended the class on stress yesterday and another on getting better sleep. I also have a book I am supposed to read for work called, *Stop Stress this Minute*. But honestly, what helps me most is just going to my happy place. Surely, you have one too. Where does your mind go in between tasks? Where does it go when you punch the clock to go home? Some people have to go outside. Some people have to go to the ocean or the bar or the shoe store or the TV. I don't really need to GO anywhere, but I think about friends that are dear to me. I think about what fun thing is next on my schedule. (Anticipation is way underrated.) Lately, I am thinking about building. I think about how amazingly blessed I am.

And often I think about the one thinking about me:

Psalm 48:9

Within your temple, O God, we meditate on your unfailing love.

Whether near or far, you are often my happy place. Love, Lynn

Working With, Not Against

October 19, 2013

I am writing early this morning because I have plenty to share even though my day just started. I shared with you on Wednesday that I was feeling the physical results of stress in my body. Thursday I shared how I was dealing with stress by setting my mind to think differently. Yesterday, I had another good, productive day at work, but I could still feel the muscle tension in my back and neck. I thought surely, if I can just make it to yoga, I can work all that out and get back to normal. We worked really hard in yoga, but it didn't work. I thought, well, of course, I will just get to bed and in the morning I will be fine. I woke this morning with neck pain and then the headache I have been waiting to happen blossomed, finding its way up the back of my neck into the base of my head and then around to my brow and forehead.

Before Gerson therapy I suffered from two kinds of pain, headaches and menstrual cramps and for 35 years I dealt with both the same way. Just give me a can of Diet Coke and 3 or 4 Ibuprofen. That should take care of it. And if it doesn't, well, just hand me another Coke. Max Gerson has a different prescription altogether. One coffee enema, 500 MG of vitamin C, 50 MG of Niacin and one adult aspirin. So, I forced myself out of bed and started. Of course when I used the little girl's room, I discovered I have my period.

I have said time and time again that I want to recognize the cycles of my life and the cycles of my body so that I can work with them and not against them. I have made great progress, making the most of sleep cycles, making the most of regulated eating times, learning to respect my body and natural laws in those ways. However, my hatred for my menstrual cycle has resulted in more childish behavior. I keep trying to will it away, try to ignore the fact that it will show up, deny that I have to be subject to the powerful influences and effects on my emotional and physical being, trying to power through, previously, on Coke and drugs.

All this stuff this week, I now attribute to my cycle. Had I acknowledged that cycle and respected its effects maybe I could have prepared, maybe I could have anticipated and spent a little more time in a quiet space, a meditative space. Maybe I could have worked to protect my schedule a little better, to set my mind. Powering through on Coke and Ibuprofen is not only not an option any longer, it was not a wise strategy in the first place. I need to work with the laws of my body, not against.

You are wondering, does Gerson's "Pain Triad" as he called it work? My head hurt enough to want to stay in bed for sure, but the pain triad absolutely took the edge off so that I can function for the day and do what I need to do and hopefully what I want to do.

So, not Ibuprofen, but I be drug free! (except for aspirin and maybe a little organic dark chocolate)

For sure, you raise my serotonin levels! Love, Lynn

Juiced

October 20, 2013

Juicing, is that street vernacular for taking steroids? Well, anyway, I'm juicing and have been for a while. As a Christian, I find myself collecting Bibles. You would think a person only needs one. They all say the same thing. I don't know how many I have right now, 6, not sure. I find myself leaning toward that same propensity with juicers. I started with a Nutribullet. When I started Gerson therapy, I bought a Norwalk. When I didn't have time for the Norwalk, I got a Fusion. Mom doesn't like the white one and wanted a black one so we just got a black one. We were in a couple stores yesterday and we kept finding ourselves looking at the new Jack LaLane juicer that happens to look just like the Fusion. Not sure why we both keep looking. My mom is a hoarder by nature. I am a collector by nature. I think we are in trouble.

Absolutely juiced about my opportunity to love you!! Lynn

Operant Conditioner

October 23, 2013

I took a mental health day from work today. I was focusing on some reading provided by my company as part of our wellness programs. The book I read is called, *Stop Stress this Minute*. I like it. It has great info in it. It lists 8 things you can do when stressed:

Breathe
Relax
Take Inventory
Focus
Meditate
Visualize
Deep Relaxation
Vigorous Exercise

I was reading about meditating and have read many times that I should choose a mantra of some kind, a word or phrase to help me focus while I am meditating. This has been challenging for me. I have tried different words and none have really stuck. I really like the word, "healing" and keep going back to that, but I realized today, that some words for me are not good to use because even though I am saying the word in my mind, I am still using muscles in my mouth to say the word. When I say "healing" in my head, I actually move my tongue to the roof of my mouth to get the "L" sound.

I guess that is why "Om" works well. So I thunk and I thunk and finally decided on, "Ah." This works, "Ah" as in this is so relaxing and "Ah" as in yes, I understand. That's what I need, enlightened relaxation! But, I also read that if I keep using this word, it will become an operant conditioner. Yeah, I didn't know what that was either, but the author mentioned Pavlov's dogs. The bell was the operant conditioner. When the dogs heard the bell, they began to salivate because they knew the food was coming. I already associate "Ah" with relaxation so this should work well. The more I connect "Ah" with meditation, the better my practice will become.

So, of course, I tried it. The first 5 minutes didn't work at all. The second 5 minutes worked fairly well. Then I fell asleep. I know. I am supposed to meditate sitting up. Maybe someday I will use meditation to actually meditate and not just put myself to sleep.

Ahhhh, meditating on all your beautiful qualities! Love, Lynn

The Location of Opportunity

October 25, 2013

Author Stephen Covey says that all your opportunity for personal growth lies in the small space between stimulus and response. This is a great idea to ponder. What he is saying, as we have heard 100 times, is, "It is not how you act, but how you react." Specifically, in this case, how you react to events that typically cause you stress.

We can think that we have no control over how we react to events in our lives. In fact, we can. We have the power. The challenge is believing we have the power. A preacher made an excellent point one time, saying that people who claim that they have a problem with anger and just can't help but yell at their wife or kids, amazingly have all kinds of power to not ever explode at their boss. People have control over how they act and react. They just have to choose that control.

Yes, the opportunity for growth, for change, for progress, lies in that space between an event and the time it takes to react. The location is not necessarily in our brain, but in our conscience, maybe just below the surface.

Everything we know, all our experiences, all our book knowledge and all that we have seen on TV or in real life, all our dreams, our desires, our failings, our hopes and all our fears fill that tiny little space between action and reaction.

In yoga, we spend one and a half hours trying to create space in our bodies. Between events, seemingly stressful events, and our reactions, we can tap into that space in time and in the recesses of our core being and ask some simple questions.

How would I normally react in this situation? What in my beliefs, the way I understand life, makes me react that way? Did my actions bring about my desired results? Is there something I can do differently, right here, right now, that will bring about a different and better outcome? Do I need to think differently about something, change my perspective, to help me react in a more constructive way?

I'm going to start asking these questions and see if I can't find that location of opportunity.

Tapping into the recesses of my mind, where thoughts of you reside. Love you lots! Lynn

A Gerson Day

November 4, 2013

Tomorrow marks 6 months on Gerson therapy! Yippee! However, it feels like 6 years and I'm only a quarter of the way there!!! Yikes! Okay, I will focus on the accomplishment, not on the road ahead. So, I want to share with you what a normal day for me looks like:

Up at 4:45. I went downstairs and pulled a bag out of the fridge. This bag held the ingredients of one green drink. I rinsed everything in the sink and cut the apple, scooping out the seeds inside and then put everything into a plastic basket. I juiced in the Fusion juicer and then took the drink to my supplement station. I got 7 pills and added 3 iodine drops to my drink. I drank it down, swallowing the pills down too.

I went back upstairs and turned on a little heater sitting by the sink. In front of the heater was an 8 ounce mason jar with distilled water and an 8 ounce mason jar with cooked coffee. I removed the metal lids so as not to burn my hands on them after the liquids were heated. I just kept the heater on for about 5 minutes. I just want the liquids to be lukewarm. I started with a quick water enema. Then I did a coffee enema for 15 minutes. I used a yoga mat and a towel on the bathroom floor and covered myself with a heavy bath towel.

After I was finished I went back downstairs, where Mom had already juiced carrot juice and apple juice for the day. I took a cold baked potato from the fridge and put it in the NuWave oven to heat. I turned on my infrared stove top to cook my organic oatmeal and raisins that had been soaking overnight in distilled water, of course. Mom juiced my second green drink and I drank it down with a vitamin D3, a Niacin tablet and a couple liver pills. Back upstairs to shower and dress and back downstairs for my 3rd green drink and oatmeal.

At 11:00 I pulled out my Thermos' at work and had carrot and apple juice with more iodine. At 12:00, another drink and my lukewarm potato, nothing on it. By the time I left work I had finished the juice in my two Thermos' and also eaten the organic Honey Crisp apple I brought with me.

I had to stop on the way home to get some apples and carrots. I had plundered Whole Foods after church on Sunday, stocking up on greens. At Stop N' Shop I bought 15 pounds of carrots and 12 pounds of Gala apples. That will last me a few days, $45.90.

When I got home, I put away the apples and carrots in the fridge in the basement. That fridge holds only apples and carrots. There was a package on the door step. I opened it to find 3 bottles of potassium compound salts, 2 bottles of iodine drops and 2 bottles of enzymes for my tummy, $88.95.

I have been without potassium salts for a week or so, so I opened a bottle and dissolved in a quart of distilled water and placed with my supplements and then opened and mixed a second bottle, mixed and packed in my tote bag to take to work tomorrow.

Mom had already cleaned and cut the carrots for tomorrow, but I prepare the green drinks myself. I took 3 small baskets and lined them with plastic grocery bags. From the fridge I got for each basket, an apple, a little red cabbage, celery, a quarter of a green bell pepper. I stacked them and walked out to the garage where the greens fridge is. I placed in each basket a little of each: baby spinach, Bok Choy, baby romaine, red leaf lettuce, hearts of romaine, the most beautiful purple kale, collard greens, red Swiss chard and escarole.

I took each bag and tied them up and put them in the fridge in the kitchen for tomorrow.

I then started to heat what I call my un-soup. I just don't like a lot of liquid. I made it on Saturday: sweet potato, onion, garlic, cauliflower and tomato, all organic. I heated on the stove top so I ran upstairs and began warming my water and coffee. Back downstairs to eat my un-soup and drink my second carrot drink since returning home. Back upstairs for my second round of enemas. After a half hour of that, on to Caring Bridge.

I should do a third enema, but I read that you should only do them every 4 hours. Therefore, I won't have time to do another before I go to bed. Running errands is tricky that way. I got out of work 20 minutes late and had to stop for carrots and apples. If I want to do 3 enemas in the day I really need to get home and get going by 4:30. That didn't happen today.

You may also notice that a lot of the greens in my drink are not in the Gerson recipe. That's correct.

Yeah, I know. It is a long entry! I'll do what I have to do to be healthy for me and you!! Love, Lynn

Six Months!

November 5, 2013

Well here it is! Six months on Gerson therapy! A milestone indeed. Today, I was buried at work with a long to do list in front of me and I thought, "Yeah, but I am accomplishing great things on Gerson" and I smiled on the inside.

Of course, none of this would even matter if you hadn't been here all along to help me through, giving me the privilege to share with you every day, long winded or short.

Okay, 180 days down and only 550 to go. Keep smiling Lynn!

Thanks for climbing this mountain with me! Lots of love!

Process Improvement for 2014

November 6, 2013

When we, alright, when I was a kid I could learn a thing or two by watching TV commercials. For instance, Wonder Bread would help me grow in 12 ways!! And Keds' PF Flyer sneakers would make me, "run faster and jump higher." Who doesn't want to run faster and jump higher? That purchase would be an important process improvement for a kid on the playground or on the dodge ball court.

I still want to run faster and jump higher. That means I'm always looking for process improvement, always looking for ways to reach new heights. Gerson therapy requires me to use my brain, to look for better, faster, less expensive ways to do things. It has been like a fun game. So far, I think I'm winning!

I'm so grateful you are playing this game of life with me!! Love, Lynn

I Dunno

November 9, 2013

Today I made it back to my yoga class. We had a substitute instructor this morning and I was so grateful to be in her class. Her name is Ann and class was at Dragonfly Studio in Marshfield. She could see that we didn't all know what we were doing and she let us know, in a very polite way of course. I have only been practicing yoga a little more than two years, maybe three, so I still have to look at my neighbors to see what they do when the instructor says a pose using the Indian name. My brain seems to reject actually remembering the Indian name with the pose. However, I have literally done the same poses hundreds of times and I thought I have been doing them correctly, as far as my body is able.

I can just go through life not knowing what I don't know. And, the more I learn, the more I learn that I don't know. The quality of my life is always richer when I am learning. My parents did not ask every night at the kitchen table, "What did you learn at school today?" They asked, "Is your homework done." School was about finishing and getting it done, not so much about learning and growing. I have read more than once that you when you stop learning, you stop having fun. I don't know if that is entirely true, but I do know that when I am learning, I'm having fun!

Proverbs 1:7

The fear of the Lord is the beginning of knowledge,

I dunno what I would do without knowledge of you! Much love, Lynn

Some Things Never Change

November 10, 2013

I was reminded of a story today, a story about a man named Naaman. I love the Bible because even though I read about people who lived 2000 years ago, people were the same then as they are today.

Naaman was a man of great status and prestige, but he contracted leprosy. A servant girl in his household told him to go to the prophet Elisha and he would be healed. He took that advice, but look at what happened when he got there:

2 Kings 5:9-12

So Naaman went with his horses and chariots and stopped at the door of Elisha's house. Elisha sent a messenger to say to him, "Go, wash yourself seven times in the Jordan, and your flesh will be restored and you will be cleansed."

But Naaman went away angry and said, "I thought that he would surely come out to me and stand and call on the name of the Lord his God, wave his hand over the spot and cure me of my leprosy. Are not Abana and Pharpar, the rivers of Damascus, better than all the waters of Israel? Couldn't I wash in them and be cleansed?" So he turned and went off in a rage.

Naaman had a preconceived idea about how he should be healed. And when it wasn't what he expected, he was insulted and angry. His pride got in the way. He eventually did what Elisha told him to do and was healed.

Are we not exactly the same way? If we contract a serious illness we expect someone to say, "Hey, I can get you an appointment with this world renowned specialist in the best, cutting edge hospital in Boston. This guy is impossible to get an appointment with, but he owes me a favor so he is willing to see you."

So when a 90 year old woman who doesn't even have a medical degree tells us, just juice and by the way learn to get comfortable on the bathroom floor, we think she is out of her mind. There is no way that could work. If it worked, everyone would be doing it. Hey, you can wash yourself in the River Dana-Farber or the River Beth Israel or whatever river you want. I'll be down at the River Gerson, dipping seven times. In this case Max Gerson was the prophet and daughter Charlotte is just the messenger. I'm all ears.

No problem, I'll hang with you in the leper colony! Lots of love, Lynn

Gerson Gray

November 12, 2013

I am not supposed to color my hair on Gerson therapy because of the chemicals. You might think, "Okay, so what's the big deal? Don't color your hair." Others of you might be thinking, "What?? Are you crazy? I would have to color my hair." I have been using the most natural stuff I can find at Whole Foods. I have been coloring my hair for around 10 years. I know how to follow the directions on the box. Yet, I colored it recently and the gray was showing through in no time. I colored it again just before Halloween and the gray is already back.

I'm seriously thinking of just surrendering at this point. Hey, I'll save $18.00 a month. That is equal to 3 bags or 9 pounds of organic apples! The only reason I color is to appease my own ego. There really is no important reason to color. I think my biggest concern is, not that people will think I'm old, but maybe that people will think I'm too sick to care for myself or they may think I've lost my mind, gone all crazy on Gerson. Plus, I honestly cannot visualize what I would look like with gray hair.

Some reasons are floating in my head why maybe I shouldn't go gray. What if I apply for a loan at a bank? Am I going to look to old to pay off the mortgage? What if I have to interview for a job? Are they going to want someone younger or younger looking? Hmmmm...things to think about, I guess.

I'll love you in any color you choose! Lynn

Only What I Can Bear

November 13, 2013

When I started Gerson therapy, it was super challenging. After a month or so, I was getting used to it. When I went back to work it was super tough. Now, I'm in a groove for the most part, plus I have a super hero accomplice, Mom. That helps! Then the house started getting colder inside and I had to make adjustments in the bathroom, smaller mason jars and now using a heater.

NOW, it is getting colder outside. I'm so grateful I was able to begin Gerson therapy in May. The outside was not only forgiving, but encouraging. But things are changing and how. I went out to the garage tonight to prepare my green drinks for tomorrow. My fingers were frozen by the time I was done. I've considered pulling out all the ingredients at once, but there is absolutely no room to put them down anywhere. I could get rubber gloves and wear those thin winter gloves underneath...maybe. I could turn the heat on in the garage, no, massively expensive, or we could put a larger fridge in the basement, possibly switch the small fridge in the basement with the big fridge in the garage. Just not sure.

The other challenge is going out to shop. Its only November and it was freezing today. I looked on line at Pea Pod delivery service. The website says they don't deliver to my zip code, naturally.

If you don't have to work and you are going to start Gerson therapy, find a friend who lives in the south who has large capacity fridges and a guest suite with a private bathroom. Then you'll be fine!

1 Corinthians 10:13

No temptation has overtaken you except what is common to mankind. And God is faithful; he will not let you be tempted beyond what you can bear....like the temptation to bail on Gerson :)

I am never tempted to bail on you! Lots of love, Lynn

Live Victoriously!

November 14, 2013

This is not so much my motto as a directive to myself each day. When I start to feel like I'm not handling my daily challenges well, or overcoming obstacles or I begin to allow myself to feel NOT victorious; I tell myself, "Live victoriously!" Does it help? I think so. A friend commented on Gerson Girl the other day after reading my story, "I guess that is why sometimes you are so forceful and I mean that in a good way." For me, it takes being forceful, mostly with myself, to live victoriously.

It does not take much to be defeated or to feel defeated on any given day. So much comes at us. So much can derail our mission, whatever that mission or goal is that day. Physical limitations, time constraints, demands on our brains, on our emotions, needs pulling at us, our own desires and wants or our own weaknesses and failings. It's amazing to me that we even make it through a day whole. AND I've got it easy! I don't have a spouse or children or elderly parents that I have to care for or please or appease. In fact, I have an elderly parent caring for me.

I was battling one of those weaknesses today and have been for some time. I have been dipping into the candy bowl AGAIN at work. Finally, I remembered that when I first got my diagnosis, I had turned to a verse that helped me gain some conviction:

2 Corinthians 7:1

Therefore, since we have these promises, dear friends, let us purify ourselves from everything that contaminates body and spirit, perfecting holiness out of reverence for God.

I have already won the victory, having you in my life!! Lots of love, Lynn

My Super Hero

November 15, 2013

I was talking to my other super hero last night, not my mom. I dozed off before I was done speaking with him, so I will start again. I don't think he will mind if I share with you.

You are the genesis of my soul.
You are the guardian of my heartbeat.
You have numbered the hairs on my head
and my days on the earth.
You wake me with a fiery star
and usher me to sleep with a lantern in the sky.
You hug me through a thousand arms
and kiss me through a thousand lips
You hedge me in, on every side

with love, compassion, mercy and comfort.
You lift me up with words, ever so powerful words!
You lived for me and you've died for me.
You are everything to me. I am nothing without you.
Because I see a glimpse of how you see,
Everyone else is radiant too!
Yes, the genesis of my soul and the holder of the key,
the key to my eternal destiny.
My creator, my husband and my God.
I love you and I belong to you!

Yes indeed, when I look at you I see radiance! Love, Lynn

Imagine That!

November 16, 2013

A year or so ago, a minister in our church fellowship came to town to do a one man dramatic presentation about the apostle John. The proceeds would go to support an alternative therapy for his sick wife Lisa. This was a therapy not covered by their insurance company. Later, when I was diagnosed and looking into Gerson therapy I wondered if Lisa was doing Gerson therapy, but I didn't know her personally so I never found out. My friend Emily had worshipped with Lisa in New York and recently asked me if I was doing the same treatment as Lisa. I responded that I didn't know. Emily mentioned the doctor Lisa had seen in NY, Nick Gonzalez MD, a famous immunologist.

Last Sunday a woman, Mary, in church asked, "Are you juicing?" I said I was. She said, "I worked for a top immunologist in New York. I've seen him cure cancer with juicing." I ran into Mary again tonight. She said, "I worked for Nick Gonzalez." Mary told me that he heals with juicing, coffee enemas and organic foods. His training was in New York under someone, I think who must have been super familiar with Gerson therapy. Gerson practiced in New York in the 30s and 40s.

"Nicholas J. Gonzalez, MD - He received his medical degree from Cornell University Medical College, New York City, in 1983. During a postgraduate immunology fellowship under Robert A. Good, MD, PhD, considered the father of modern Immunology and for years President of Sloan-Kettering, he completed a research study evaluating an aggressive nutritional therapy in the treatment of advanced cancer. Since 1987, Dr. Gonzalez has been in private practice in New York City, treating patients diagnosed with cancer and other serious degenerative illnesses."

Huh! Imagine that! Loving you! Lynn

Mammogram?

Nov 17, 2013

A coworker said she was going for her mammogram after work the other day. I said that I might opt not to have a mammogram. She looked at me curiously. I said that, well, I'm doing Gerson therapy. If I'm doing Gerson therapy, I shouldn't have breast cancer. I could see she was thinking about it.

Does Gerson therapy work on some cancer and not others? As noted in, *Healing the Gerson Way*, there are some cancers that are tough to cure with Gerson therapy. Brain cancer is tough because the normally healing inflammation can cause headaches or seizures in a swelling brain. Bone metastases is challenging because it is painful and takes a very long time to heal, open breast cancer lesions, some leukemia, multiple myeloma, disease in anybody who has had long term steroid or chemo treatment. These are all tough to heal with Gerson, but can be healed.

That said, does it make sense to subject myself to a mammogram? If they find cancer, what would I do? Could I defeat bladder cancer and still have another cancer show up some place else? That might be possible, but I would think highly improbable.

Am I super woman? Not by any stretch of the imagination. Am I being arrogant to think I might not need routine screenings? I don't know. I don't think so.

Everything is ruled by science. I think if I do what I am supposed to do, most of the time, and get adequate rest, the science that has defeated my bladder cancer will continue to create a hostile environment to cancer every place else in my body. I guess time will tell.

Conversely, desiring to create a warm and welcoming environment for you! Lots of love! Lynn

Kevin's Story

November 19, 2013

I can't tell you all the details, but I will tell you what I know. My brother works with Kevin. Kevin is I'm guessing in his late 40s or in his 50s. He was recently diagnosed with pancreatic cancer. I've met him once. He has been curing himself with food and detoxing. I asked him if he was doing Gerson therapy. He said he had read the book. I asked him if he was juicing. His response was, "Not as much as you are." I asked him, well I didn't, but he does not do coffee enemas. He does however go to the Internal Wellness Center in Dedham for colon cleansing. He was diagnosed probably more than a year ago. He has not done any treatment prescribed by his doctors. His cancer seems to be gone. He is working full days, full time. All symptoms appear to be gone. I don't know if he has been tested to see if indeed it is all gone.

Kevin is not on the Gerson diet, specifically. He is not on the Gerson juicing regimen. He has created for himself an obviously, liberally modified form of Gerson therapy and for him it is working. The tricky part with modified Gerson, is you never know where the tipping point in your battle is. How much can you modify before the therapy just doesn't work?

The good news is that there is promise for anyone, to do what you can, even if you can't do it all, every day. If you want to do Gerson and are feeling like I did, thinking there is no way I can do this the way I need to, then I say dive in anyway. You won't drown. You will learn how to swim and get through.

For anyone who needs it, and who doesn't! Sending you bucket loads of hope and determination for the ride or swim, whatever your challenge. Love you lots! Lynn

Guest Writer -Janet Stillings

November 22, 2013

I am grateful and delighted to share some words from Janet Stillings, wife of Dr. Donald Stillings of *The Longevity Center*, now located in the Midwest. She is also the one who cooked every bite for me during my 10 day visit. She juiced every juice and measured out all my supplements. I'm grateful I had the chance to meet and know her.

My name is Janet Stillings and I have been co-laboring with Dr. Stillings to teach and deliver the Gerson Therapy to many people over the past twelve years. I feel blessed to participate in supporting those interested in seeking an alternative, holistic approach for the healing of their chronic and degenerative conditions. Though it is often not a first choice for many and definitely not an easy one, allowing and cooperating with the body to heal itself is an amazing journey. As Psalm 139:14 so aptly puts it, "I will praise You, for I am awesomely and wonderfully made." Why not take this conservative choice as a first choice instead of a last resort and see what your body can do?

Our program guarantees that your body will experience no harm. It is gentle and safe. It invades your system with live foods, flooding your internal parts with all manner of goodness. It detoxifies the liver mainly through coffee enemas thereby flushing the system of harmful, built up toxins. Through this flooding and flushing process, your body is given the ability to recreate and realign its internal environment from a state of weakness and illness to one of vitality and wellness. It must be understood this goal is not accomplished overnight which becomes a real challenge for our concepts today that demand an easy, quick fix. It's hard to imagine that since we became ill over a period of time, the laws of biology dictate that it will take time to heal. It's difficult to take responsibility for the abuse we rendered to our body, that it would have repercussions. Perhaps, we need to consider giving ourselves time to heal as we "fight the good fight" to work with our body instead of against it.

Again, I am grateful to be part of a work that aligns with our organic, innate, God given abilities. I am thankful to have touched and been able to serve in a small way the lives of many extraordinary people. Lynn Ford is such a person.

Janet is an angel and a very hard working one at that, a hero, leading the way in the education of the people, the people who need it most, in Gerson therapy. She is there at a tenuous time in people's lives, a pivotal moment between wellness and illness, even life and death.

Much thanks to you Janet and God bless you for your service in his name. Love, Lynn

Gerson Grit

November 24, 2013

Usually when I am trying to describe what Gerson therapy is like, I use the word "rigorous." I think that is a pretty good fit. But I think too that Gerson therapy is making me tougher than I was. I can be lazy. I can be undisciplined. I can be neglectful of my body. I can procrastinate. Gerson therapy does not allow for any of those things. Ten or eleven hours a day, I have to do something Gerson. This Gerson Grit I am developing is helping me be more mindful of how I spend every minute. It helps me be Not lazy. It helps me be Not undisciplined, Not neglectful of my body, Not procrastinating.

It is so easy to listen to the 5 year old inside when I am faced with a choice or as I like to say, 1000 choices, in a day. She immediately voices her opinion and it is always the same. "I don't wanna." And I reply back, "Sometimes we have to do things we don't like," or more recently, "Do the things you HAVE to SO THAT you can do the things you WANT to." That quiets her till the next uneasy task. Occasionally she tugs on my shirt, "May of 2015? That's too long. I can't do this that long." I just smile lovingly and say, "We can do it. We've come this far. One day at a time." Then she settles for a time.

Sometimes, there is just no room for, "I don't wanna." Here's that funny passage about Paul's, "I don't wanna."

Romans 7:14-20

We know that the law is spiritual; but I am unspiritual, sold as a slave to sin. I do not understand what I do. For what I want to do I do not do, but what I hate I do. And if I do what I do not want to do, I agree that the law is good. As it is, it is no longer I myself who do it, but it is sin living in me. For I know that good itself does not dwell in me, that is, in my sinful nature. For I have the desire to do what is good, but I cannot carry it out. For I do not do the good I want to do, but the evil I do not want to do—this I keep on doing. Now if I do what I do not want to do, it is no longer I who do it, but it is sin living in me that does it.

I just wanna thank God for you! Love, Lynn

Guest Writer – Lisa Burgess

December 2, 2013

Guest writer Lisa Burgess is gracing us with her wisdom. Lisa is a sweet, Godly woman from Huntsville AL. She has been blogging for many years and just started on Facebook under, *Lisa's Notes…on Seeing God*. She writes:

We've all heard of post-traumatic stress disorder (PTSD), the haunting anxiety after a severe trauma. But have you heard of post-traumatic growth (PTG)? It's just as real.

Research in PTG ramped up in the 1990s, defining it as "positive psychological change experienced as a result of struggle with highly challenging life circumstances." But trace it back further to Romans 8:28, "And we know that for those who love God all things work together for good, for those who are called according to his purpose."

We can look at Lynn for proof. Instead of reacting to a cancer diagnosis with passive hopelessness, Lynn looked up to God, looked out to others, and looked in for change, adjusting her thinking and her behaviors to new facts and conditions.

Three areas of change are most documented among PTG:

1. Change in perceptions of self (as a survivor, a greater sense of strength),

2. Change in relationships with others (more open, more giving), and

3. Change in philosophy of life (different priorities, great appreciation for life).

It's not just returning to "normal," to how you were before the event, but instead, by the grace of God, coming out stronger.

Do we have to go through trauma to experience this? No. But getting closer to dying often wakes us up more fully to living. Even if you're crisis-free at the moment, you know someone else in pain. Hang out together. Learn from them. Pray for their growth. Not only can you help them get stronger, you may come out stronger, too. To God be the glory.

Thank you Lisa!! Much love from Boston!

...And feeling much love in Boston from all of you, Lynn

Ridiculous!

December 19, 2013

Just had to write. On ABC news last night, they said that 10 of the last 12 cancer drugs approved by the FDA cost over $100,000 a year.

How's Gerson therapy sound now?

These drugs don't cure cancer. They just keep the cancer at bay as long as you pay for the drugs. I mean, as long as you use the drugs.

How's Gerson therapy sound now?

They also stated that people with a cancer diagnosis are twice as likely to go bankrupt as people without a cancer diagnosis.

How's Gerson therapy sound now?

Gee, I guess $2 a pound for organic apples isn't so bad after all.

Willing to pay most any price for your continued love! Lynn

In Conclusion

It is January 22, 2014 as I write this last entry. I am in my 8th month of Gerson therapy. I have 16 more months to go. You may ask why I am stopping my book here? I anticipate the next 16 months to be much of the same as the last 8. I am still receiving medical treatment for bladder cancer even though there was no cancer to be seen on September 4th. The protocol, depending on which hospital I go to, calls for 2 to 3 years of BCG maintenance. Since September 4th I have had 3 more BCG treatments. I went for a scope on January 21st to see if anything has changed, to see if any cancer has returned. I was pretty confident all would be well, but I have also learned that I cannot take for granted the great results I am looking for. My bladder was clean as a whistle. Whew! I'm sure there are plenty of people who stop practicing Gerson therapy when they find their cancer is gone, which of course is unwise. I pray that I can keep my head and heart in the game for the duration of the 2 years Max Gerson demanded of his patients. I also want to stop here because I am eager to share what I have learned and can't wait any longer.

I am working full time and doing my best not to overdo at work. I am very protective of my sleep schedule even though good things pull at my heart. I have not travelled since starting Gerson therapy. I was wishing my young friend Anna in Alabama a happy birthday the other day on Facebook. She said, "Love you and miss you so much. Please come visit." I took care of Anna when she was just a little baby. It is hard for me to say, "Sorry, not now, not yet." I'm sure my desire to see her is greater than her desire to see me, but it is that kind of sacrifice that makes sticking to this hard sometimes. In addition, my very serious goal is to open a facility someday to share what I know with others. Making that dream come true also demands incredible sacrifice even now as I try to plan financially how to bring this dream to fruition.

This book is called, *God and Gerson Therapy*. I contemplated calling it, *Gerson Therapy with God*, but I wanted "God" to be first. The older I get and the more I understand of God, the more evident it becomes that in all things, God is first. He doesn't just want to be first, he IS first in all things whether I acknowledge that or not. I want God to be first in my life, in all my decisions and all my considerations. I totally believe that God knows what is best for my life and if I keep seeking and asking that he will show me the best ways to go at every juncture.

If you want to find me, I'm posting as "Gerson Girl" on Facebook. Please send me your feedback or questions. My hope and prayer is that you found what you were looking for and more here. I pray that you found knowledge and more importantly inspiration, courage and even faith. I pray that you find healing and health and I pray that in your walk on this road you will find deep, pure love and you will be a giver of deep, pure love. May God bless you and prosper you.

A seed must push up from beneath the earth.
Its struggle makes it strong
A tree must endure the wind
Its struggle makes it strong
For every challenge to the brain;
A math problem, learning to read, navigating an airport-
Its struggle makes it strong
A heart and mind faces many troubles
Day after day after day

…but from beneath the burden, enduring the storms, navigating events, the struggle makes them strong. Sunshine, smiling faces and the thrill and miracle of love make all the work worthwhile…XO

Other Purported Cancer Fighters

Here is just a list of foods or supplements that folks have claimed can defeat cancer. I haven't seen any studies, I haven't researched, but I just want to pass along to you so that you can have these extra weapons in your arsenal as you strive for optimal health in your own life.

Essiac : This comes in tea or pill form, from Canada. I used Essiac to compliment Gerson therapy. I did not take the full prescribed dose, maybe half.

Salvestrol: This is a plant supplement developed in England, distributed from Canada. I took this on recommendation of a Naturopath friend.

Soursop or Graviola: I have seen this on the internet and heard someone touting it. I have no more knowledge of this product.

Pau D'Arco tea: I have heard good things about this tea.

Spirulina and other algaes: for your green drink

Onions and Mushrooms: angio genesis prohibitors

My friend Maria from Argentina says the Shamans of South America have been using herbs to heal for thousands of years. Here are some things she suggests: Cat's Claw, Bitter Melon and Grape Seed

Favorite Books, Documentaries and Juicers

Documentaries:

Forks Over Knives

Food Matters

Hungry for Change

Food Inc.

Ingredients

The Gerson Miracle

Books:

The Daniel Plan by Daniel Amen, MD
Toxic Relief by Don Colbert, MD
Anti-Cancer: A New Way of Life by David Servan-Schreiber, MD, PhD (for cancer)
Eat to Live by Joel Fuhrman, MD
The Maker's Diet by Jordan Rubin
Healing the Gerson Way by Charlotte Gerson (for Cancer and other serious disease)
What are You Hungry For? by Deepak Chopra
Forks Over Knives, edited by Gene Stone
The pH Balance Diet by Vyas and LeQuesne
Super Foods by David Wolfe

Juicers:

Obviously, the Norwalk is the Gerson recommended juicer, but not everyone can buy one of those. If you are not doing Gerson therapy, a Nutribullet is good for one or two juices a day. It keeps all the fiber. You can also add nuts and seeds to a Nutribullet. For serious juicing to fight existing disease and for optimal health, I use a Fusion. I use a Fusion instead of the Norwalk because I don't have time for the Norwalk. It extracts the juice and requires much more produce per glass. The secret for a great tasting green drink – add an apple. Gerson says Granny Smith, I use Gala. When juicing, always strive for organic produce. There a tons of juicers on the market. The Nutribullet and the Fusion are about $120.00 Jack La Lane has a juicer that looks exactly like the Fusion. I like the fusion because it claims to not heat the juice, which kills the enzymes, which is important.

Not to be forgotten, consistent, moderate exercise is 20% of the health equation. If you are healthy, Ping pong is excellent at working all muscle groups and your brain as well ☺. If you are trying to heal, maybe just a 20 or 30 minute walk.